Betty Crocker's

NEW

EAT AND LOSE

WEIGHT

Betty Crocker's

NEW

EAT AND LOSE

WEIGHT

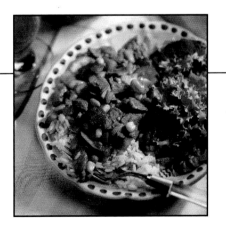

MACMILLAN   USA

MACMILLAN
A Simon & Schuster Macmillan Company
1633 Broadway
New York, NY 10019

MACMILLAN is a registered trademark of Macmillan, Inc.

BETTY CROCKER is a registered trademark of General Mills, Inc.

Library of Congress Cataloging-in-Publication

Crocker, Betty.
    [New eat and lose weight]
    Betty Crocker's new eat and lose weight.
        p.   cm.
    Includes index.
    ISBN 0-02-861500-X (alk. paper)   ISBN 0-02-862638-9 (pb)
    1. Reducing diets—Recipes.   2. Reducing exercises.
RM222.2.C754   1997
641.5'635—dc20   96-26602
                                                                         CIP

GENERAL MILLS, INC.

Betty Crocker Kitchens

Director: Marcia Copeland
Editor: Lori Fox
Recipe Development: Altanette Autry, Mary Carroll, Nancy Cooper, Anne Stuart
Food Stylists: Kate Courtney Condon, Cindy Lund
Nutritionist: Elyse A. Cohen, M.S., Nancy Holmes, R.D.
Photographer: Carolyn Luxmoore

Cover design: Iris Jeromnimon
Book design: George J. McKeon

For consistent baking results, the Betty Crocker Kitchens
recommend Gold Medal flour.

You can create great-tasting food with these approved recipes from the Betty Crocker Kitchens.
Cooking and baking have never been so easy or enjoyable!

Manufactured in the United States of America

10 9 8 7 6 5 4

First edition

Cover photo: Grilled Shrimp Kabobs (page 122)
Back cover photos: Stuffed French Toast (page 58); Creamy Vegetable-Cheese Soup (page 70);
Lemon-Filled Fresh Ginger Scones (page 65)

Introduction

Did you ever think you could eat delicious food, lose weight, and feel great—all at the same time? Well, you can! America's most loved and trusted cook shows you how with *Betty Crocker's New Eat and Lose Weight.* We've revised our very popular first edition of *Betty Crocker's Eat and Lose Weight* packed with *more* tasty and satisfying recipes using low-fat and low-calorie ingredients that are readily available in your local supermarkets. In this new edition you'll also find our Three-Step Guide to make eating and losing weight so much easier, enjoyable and rewarding.

Losing weight fits easily into your life with clear manageable steps. Our Three-Step Guide shows you how to eat smart by making healthy food choices, energizing with exercise and planning realistic, achievable goals. It's so simple—in three easy steps. All the information we've included supports your goal of losing weight with easy-to-follow charts and worksheets to help measure your progress, calorie charts to help you plan meals and sound advice to help steer you away from dieting myths and misconceptions.

Yet, the best part of *Betty Crocker's New Eat and Lose Weight* are of course the recipes! We know that the 196 recipes we've gathered here will keep you and your family truly satisfied any meal of the day. They are full of variety and great taste, ranging from delicious snacks and appetizers to tasty main dishes and luscious desserts. We know you'll love diving into a bowl of Louisiana Seafood Creole or a plate of Fettucine Carbonara, Wild Mushroom Pizza, or Caramel-Apple Bread Pudding. Sound tempting? Just think about enjoying a warm, creamy slice of golden brown Turkey Pie with a flaky rich crust just as wonderful as Grandma's pot pie—with only 3 grams of fat per serving! You won't believe you're eating "diet" food!

And to help you reach your weight loss goals, we've included two full weeks of daily menus, including snacks. The menus are flexible—choose whatever works best for you. You can mix and match meals, and we've provided the nutritional information for each meal or snack *and* for the entire day.

Trust Betty Crocker to make weight loss easier! With lots of terrific recipes and specific and helpful information, plus an easy Three-Step Guide that works, this is truly a cookbook that anyone can use and find that weight loss can be delicious and achievable at the same time.

Betty Crocker

Contents

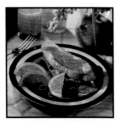
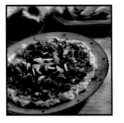
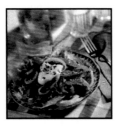
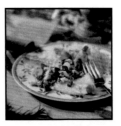
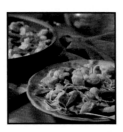

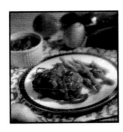
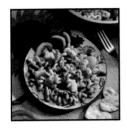
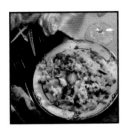
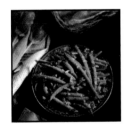
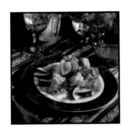

The Three-Step Guide to Losing Weight and Feeling Great!

Are you trying to lose weight and balance healthful eating with delicious food? Then we have good news! *Betty Crocker's New Eat and Lose Weight Cookbook* is just the book you have been searching for. It's packed with great-tasting recipes plus helpful information and tips to help you lose weight.

The plan is based on three easy steps to success. They are:

Step 1.   Eating Smart
Step 2.   Energize with Exercise
Step 3.   Go for the Goals

Getting Started

Before starting any weight-loss or exercise plan, first check with your doctor and get his or her approval and medical advice. Once you get the go-ahead, it is important to remember not to expect to lose lots of weight quickly. Losing one to two pounds per week is the safest and longest-lasting method for weight loss.

Building healthy lifestyle habits starts slowly at first. Experts tell us it takes three to four weeks for new habits to become automatic, and our safe and easy plan will guide you every step of the way.

Nutrition Is Important

Every recipe includes nutritional analysis and dietary exchanges. To be sure how many calories you eat each day, keep serving sizes as close as possible to what the recipe suggests. If you eat more, total calories will be higher; if you eat less, total calories will be lower. Many of the recipes are accompanied by serving suggestions, but these are not figured in the nutrition analysis.

Great-Tasting Recipes

Creating great-tasting recipes was definitely an important goal for this book. If it doesn't taste good, no matter how healthful it is, who wants to eat it? You don't have to worry about preparing separate meals for nondieting family members—these recipes are sure to please everyone.

Unbelievable, you say? If you think you can't eat some of your favorite foods and still lose weight, you'll be surprised to find out just how deliciously easy it can be to do both! How does Meat Loaf, Swiss Steak, Pork, Onion and Pepper Fajitas, Garlic Chicken Kiev, Easy Macaroni and Cheese or Scampi with Fettucine sound? Inviting, yes, flavorful, yes—fattening, no!

These recipes were developed with readily available ingredients and many of the fat-free, cholesterol-free, reduced-fat and reduced-sodium products that are available today. And, with the use of nonstick cookware, we've significantly reduced cooking fat.

Busy lifestyles can often mean we want to spend less time in the kitchen preparing meals. The majority of the recipes have eight or fewer ingredients and easy, streamlined methods of preparation and cooking. Each recipe includes preparation and cooking times to help you schedule your time in the kitchen.

Step 1: Eating Smart

The process of learning to eat smart is similar to learning how to ride a bicycle; it's wobbly at first and you need some help, but then one day, you do it all by yourself and you remember how to do it for the rest of your life.

How do you tackle the issue of losing weight? We recommend the U.S. Department of Agriculture and the U.S. Department of Health and Human Services' dietary changes to help ensure weight loss success.

- **EAT A VARIETY OF FOODS.** Balance and moderation are key to successful weight loss. Check the Food Guide Pyramid on page 13 for details about the six food groups. Write down what you eat each day to discover your eating habits, both positive and negative. Use the Daily Food Tracker on page 12 to make record keeping easier.

- **BALANCE THE FOOD YOU EAT WITH PHYSICAL ACTIVITY—MAINTAIN OR IMPROVE YOUR WEIGHT.** Many adults gain weight, increasing their risk for high blood pressure, heart disease, stroke, diabetes, certain types of cancer, arthritis, breathing problems and other illness. If you are overweight or have one of the problems mentioned above, you should try to lose weight or at least maintain your current weight.

  Heredity certainly plays a role with weight, and we cannot control that, but eating habits and exercise are two things we can control. To target a healthy weight, check the Comparison of Height and Weight and Gerontology Research Center tables on pages 26–27.

- **CHOOSE A DIET WITH PLENTY OF VEGETABLES, FRUITS AND GRAIN PRODUCTS.** This is the one area in which experts are telling us to eat more, not less!

Besides being nutritionally good for you, eating these foods also has an added bonus. They contain fiber, and some of that fiber creates bulk, which slows the rate of food absorption into the body, thereby making you feel full without overeating.

- **CHOOSE A DIET MODERATE IN SUGAR.** Foods containing high amounts of sugar are called foods with "empty calories," meaning they have no positive nutritional value. Foods high in sugar are very often high in fat and calories too. When reading labels for sugar content, be aware that sugar goes by many names, including glucose, sucrose, dextrose, maltose, lactose or fructose.

- **CHOOSE A DIET MODERATE IN SALT AND SODIUM.** All of us need sodium for proper water balance, regulating blood volume and proper functioning of our nerves and muscles. Sodium is just one of the factors affecting high blood pressure. Those individuals whose high blood pressure is sensitive to the level of salt in their diets must curtail its use. Because only a small percentage of us fit into that category and there isn't a way to predict "salt sensitivity," moderation is recommended for everyone (2,400 mg per day). The best way to reduce sodium is to use less table salt, check food labels and eat fewer salty foods such as pickles, pretzels, salted snacks, mustard, ketchup and regular soy sauce.

- **IF YOU DRINK ALCOHOLIC BEVERAGES, DO SO IN MODERATION.** Alcoholic beverages tend to be high in calories and very low in nutritional value. Alcohol can also lower inhibitions, making it that much easier to snack and overeat.

- **CHOOSE A DIET LOW IN FAT, SATURATED FAT AND CHOLESTEROL.** The average American eats almost 38% of calories from fat, which is about 84 grams of fat daily or nearly the equivalent of eating one stick of butter each day. For healthy adults, **only** 30% of calories should come from fat and no more than 10% of calories from saturated fat per day.

As for cholesterol, health experts tell us to keep dietary cholesterol intake to less than 300 milligrams each day. Cholesterol is found only in animal foods: meats, fish, poultry and dairy products. And the amount of fat that's present in these foods has no bearing on whether or not the foods contain cholesterol. It's the total amount of fat we eat, not the amount of cholesterol, that's linked to a greater risk for developing coronary heart disease and cancer.

Calorie, Fat and Cholesterol Content of Oils and Fats

Food	Unit Measure	Calories	Total Fat, g	Saturated Fat, g	Cholesterol, mg
Butter	1 tablespoon	100	12	7	30
Canola oil	1 tablespoon	120	14	1	0
Cholesterol-free reduced-calorie mayonnaise	1 tablespoon	50	5	1	0
Corn oil	1 tablespoon	120	14	2	0
Fat-free mayonnaise	1 tablespoon	10	0	0	0
Lard	1 tablespoon	120	13	5	10
Mayonnaise, soybean	1 tablespoon	100	11	2	10
Nonstick cooking spray	1 spray (2.5 seconds)	5	0	0	0
Olive oil	1 tablespoon	120	14	2	0
Solid vegetable shortening	1 tablespoon	110	13	3	0
Soybean oil	1 tablespoon	120	14	2	0
Stick corn oil margarine	1 tablespoon	100	12	2	0
Tub reduced-calorie margarine	1 tablespoon	50	6	1	0
Tub vegetable oil spread (60% fat)	1 tablespoon	80	9	2	0

Compiled by GMI from University of Minnesota Nutrition Data System, product labels and manufacturer-provided nutrition information.

Smart Food Choices

Being armed with the right information can "tip the scales" in your favor when it comes to choosing foods that have more of the good stuff and less of the not-as-good stuff. The food choice chart below will steer you in the right direction for the many food choices you make each day.

Food Choice Chart

Food Category	Choose More	Choose Less
Breads, Cereals	Whole-grain breads, whole wheat, pumpernickel, rye; bread sticks, English muffins, bagels, rice cakes, pita bread	Croissants, butter rolls
	Oat bran, oatmeal, whole-grain cereals	Presweetened cereals,
	Saltines*, pretzels*, zwieback, plain popcorn	Cheese crackers, butter crackers
Rice, Pasta	Rice, pasta	Egg noodles
Baked Goods	Angel food cake	Frosted cakes, sweet rolls, pastries, doughnuts
Fruits	Fresh, frozen or dried fruits	Fruit pies
Vegetables	Fresh or frozen vegetables	Vegetables prepared with butter, cream or cheese sauces
Meat, Poultry, Fish	Lean meats, skinless poultry, fish, shellfish	Fatty meats, organ meats, cold cuts, sausages, hot dogs
Beans, Peas	Split peas, kidney beans, navy beans, lentils, soybeans, tofu	
Eggs	Egg whites, fat-free cholesterol-free egg substitutes	Egg yolks
Milk, Cream	Skim milk, 1% milk, low-fat or fat-free buttermilk	Whole milk, 2% milk, half-and-half, whipped toppings, most nondairy creamers, sour cream
Cheese	Nonfat or low-fat cottage cheese, nonfat or low-fat cheeses, farmer cheese	Whole milk cottage cheese, hard cheeses, cream cheese
Yogurt	Nonfat or low-fat yogurt	Whole milk yogurt
Frozen Desserts	Ice milk, sherbet, nonfat or low-fat frozen yogurt	Ice cream
Fats, Oils	Polyunsaturated or monounsaturated vegetable oils: sunflower, corn, soybean, olive, safflower, sesame, canola, cottonseed	Saturated fats: coconut oil, palm oil, palm kernel oil, lard, bacon fat
Spreads	Margarine or shortening made with polyunsaturated fat	Butter
Chocolate	Cocoa	Chocolate

*Reduced-sodium varieties

Source: Adapted from The American Heart Association Diet: An Eating Plan for Healthy Americans, *American Heart Association.*

Daily Food Tracker

Date _____

By writing down what you eat each day, you get a clear picture of how you are doing. By discovering your eating patterns, you become aware of both positive and negative habits and can make changes. We recommend tracking what you eat each day for one full week. Note foods you could have eliminated with an asterisk (*).

Time	Food Eaten	Amount	Calories	Fat (g)	How I Felt	What I Was Doing and Where

Total calories = _____   **Total fat =** _____

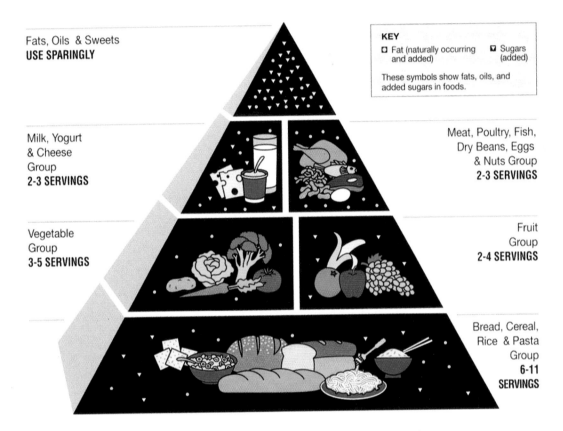

A Guide to the Food Pyramid

- The Food Guide Pyramid is divided into six parts, or food groups. Grains, the very bottom section of the pyramid, is the foundation. The idea is to eat from the bottom up, with the majority of your food choices coming from the bottom of the pyramid. The top section is Fats, Oils and Sweets, and most people need to limit their use of these foods. The five lower groups are all important, and you need food from all of them.

- Below the name of each food group are some numbers that tell you how many servings to

eat from that group each day. You need more foods from the groups at the bottom, where it is wider, than you do from the top groups.

- At each meal, serve foods from at least three different food groups. Some foods, such as tacos, combine foods from two or more different groups. Do the best you can to estimate the servings from each food group.

- It's a good idea to plan for snacks just as you plan for meals. Keep a supply of healthful snack foods on hand, such as cut-up vegetables or low-fat crackers and cookies.

Understanding Nutrition Labels

As the American lifestyle continues to quicken in pace and fewer people take time to prepare home-made foods, it becomes increasingly important to be able to read and understand the information food manufacturers provide about the nutritional content of their products. Once we learn how to read labels, we are better able to make more informed food choices.

The Nutrition Labeling and Education Act (NLEA), effective in 1994, made it mandatory by law for all packaged foods to carry a *Nutrition Facts* label. The nutrition label provides information on the nutrients we want to know more about, such as fat, saturated fat, cholesterol, sodium and fiber.

Information about nutrients is listed in grams or milligrams based on specified serving sizes derived from the amount of foods people actually eat. This way NLEA labels are standardized to make product comparisons by nutrients easier. The Percent Daily Value, a measure of how a particular food stacks up when compared to an average diet of 2,000 calories per day, is listed for certain nutrients as well.

All foods are required to list ingredients on the label in descending order of predominance by weight. For example, the *ingredient list* on a regular can of green beans might read, "Green beans, water, salt." That means that the can contains more green beans than water or salt, and more water than salt. If, however, the green beans are labeled "low sodium," they must meet the FDA guidelines for a "low sodium" product.

Health Claims: What Can Be Said

Can a diet help reduce the risk for heart disease, cancer or osteoporosis? Some food packages may now carry health claims. A health claim is a label statement that describes the relationship between a nutrient and a disease or health-related condition. A food must meet certain nutrient levels to make a health claim.

Seven types of health claims based on nutrient-disease relationships are permitted on food packages and are listed below.

LABEL HEALTH CLAIMS

A diet that is:	May help to reduce the risk of:
High in calcium	Osteoporosis (brittle bone disease)
High in fiber-containing grain products, fruits and vegetables	Cancer
High in fruits or vegetables (high in dietary fiber or vitamins A or C)	Cancer
High in fiber from fruits, vegetables and grain products	Heart disease
Low in fat	Cancer
Low in saturated fat and cholesterol	Heart disease
Low in sodium	High blood pressure (hypertension)

Nutrition Claims: What They Mean

The government also set standard definitions for terms used to describe product claims, such as *light, low fat* and *high fiber*. Now we can better understand the meaning of these claims and trust what we read on packages and in advertising. These claims can only be used if a food meets strict government definitions. Here are some of the meanings:

LABEL NUTRITION CLAIMS

Label Claim	Definition (per serving)
Low Calorie	40 calories or less
Light or Lite	1/3 fewer calories *or* 50 percent less fat than the original product; if more than half the calories are from fat, fat content must be reduced by 50 percent or more
Light in Sodium	50 percent less sodium
Fat Free	Less than 0.5 gram of fat
Low Fat	3 grams of fat or less
Cholesterol Free	Less than 2 milligrams of cholesterol and 2 grams or less saturated fat
Low Cholesterol	20 milligrams or less cholesterol and 2 grams or less saturated fat
Sodium Free	Less than 5 milligrams sodium
Very Low Sodium	35 milligrams or less sodium
Low Sodium	140 milligrams or less sodium
High Fiber	5 grams or more of fiber

Walking the Thin Line: Eating Disorders

Striving to be slim in a society that equates being thin with being popular and attractive is a concern more prevalent among young women, but affects young men as well. One unfortunate result of this pressure is that the number of young people, especially women, suffering from eating disorders is on the rise.

Although medical descriptions of eating disorders date from several centuries, little attention has focused on them until recently. The disorders usually strike people between fifteen and twenty who have a distorted attitude about eating and body image. Anorexia nervosa, one of the disorders, is described as an excessive weight loss, sometimes to the point of starvation and death. Another disorder, bulimia nervosa, is characterized by bingeing—eating very large amounts of food in short periods of time—followed by a regular pattern of self-induced vomiting, obsession with exercise or laxative abuse and fasting.

Why some are more susceptible than others to societal pressures to be thin is not known. Scientists are trying to determine the causes of eating disorders but believe both body and mind seem to play a role and are important in treatment. If a family member or friend suffers from an eating disorder, seek medical help at once. Many hospitals have eating disorder clinics and independent eating disorder clinics exist as well.

To help keep things in perspective for growing young people, encourage high self-esteem, healthful eating habits and regular exercise.

Dubious Diets

We've been bombarded with new fad diets that make big promises, but beware, many of those diets are not considered safe. Below we've described the pitfalls of some of the most popular diets.

FAD DIETS

The Diet	The Concerns
Low-calorie Diets: (under 1,200 calories per day) Limited amounts of food, especially protein, complex carbohydrates and fat.	• RDA guidelines for daily nutrients often are not met. • Although weight loss is often two to three pounds per week, it is mostly water weight and gaining it back is more likely than with slower loss diets.
High Carbohydrate and High Fiber Diets: Whole grains, cereals, raw fruits and vegetables, some protein and dairy products. Highly processed foods are discouraged.	• High amounts of fiber may reduce the absorption of minerals.
Liquid Diets: Powders and liquids are consumed as a meal replacement.	• Most people quit due to lack of variety. • Healthful eating habits are not established. • Can cause constipation. • May cause menstrual problems if calorie level is too low. • Due to the large amounts of water lost with *very low calorie* liquid diets, when normal eating is resumed, the body compensates by retaining massive amounts of fluid, which can dilute the body's potassium, causing abnormal heart rhythms. • Use of these products is safer if used daily for one meal only along with two meals of regular foods.
High Protein Diets: High protein foods such as chicken and cottage cheese are emphasized.	• Can increase levels of blood fat and cholesterol. • May cause menstrual problems. • Dehydration. • Osteoporosis. • Aggravation of gout. • Kidney stones or kidney failure.
Single Food Diets: Only one type of food such as grapefruit or rice is allowed.	• RDA guidelines for daily nutrients often are not met or are excessive in some areas. • Most people quit due to lack of variety. • Healthful eating habits are not established.
Fasting: Water and any beverages without calories are allowed.	• RDA guidelines for daily nutrients often are not met. • Low blood pressure. • Emotional disturbances. • Death if prolonged. • Healthful eating habits are not established.

DIET GIMMICKS

Diet gimmicks do not melt away extra weight and they can be costly. The safety of many gimmicks could be an issue. If losing weight were that easy, we'd be a nation of very slender people.

- Patches applied to the skin that promise to melt fat while you sleep and burn fat all day long, without vigorous exercise.

- Weight loss garments such as shorts that promise weight loss and cellulite elimination without dieting or exercise.

- Cookies and wafers that promise to melt pounds away.

- Scented pens that tell your brain you've just eaten food, so you won't gain weight.

- Food supplements/pills that melt away fat while you sleep.

- One-day diets that alternate fasting with special nutrient pills and wafers and pigging out.

- Creams and lotions that melt away fat.

- Juices/teas that make you drop the weight.

- Breath sprays that curb all your food cravings.

- Large newspaper or magazine ads that announce new medical breakthroughs that shed pounds fast without dieting. These often state that these breakthroughs are supported by doctors and professional institutions.

A daily program of a healthy, well-balanced diet and regular exercise is what works—there are no overnight, instant or magic cures for weight loss.

Step 2: Energize with Exercise

Paddling a canoe against a strong current can be done, but it will definitely take you longer to get to your destination. So it is with the relationship between weight loss and exercise. You can lose weight without regular exercise, but you won't lose as much, it won't happen as quickly and the weight loss won't be maintained as long.

For overall health benefits and general fitness, experts recommend exercising three to five times per week, with each session lasting twenty to thirty minutes. The twenty- to thirty-minute portion of the activity should be aerobic or cardiovascular at your target heart rate, preceded by a five-minute warm-up and followed by a five-minute cool-down. When trying to lose weight however, it is more effective to exercise five times per week and increase the time to forty-five minutes to one hour.

Exercise that involves the entire body is the most helpful for weight loss, and many forms of exercise meet that objective. Walking, swimming and bicycling are good exercises for beginners or for those who have not exercised for some time.

Whatever exercise you choose, make sure it one that you really enjoy so it will become a part of a healthful lifestyle. As with starting any regular exercise, check with your doctor first.

Keep track of your daily exercise using the Daily Exercise Tracker on page 22 and Calories Burned in Various Physical Activities table on pages 20–21.

36 Key Questions: The Right Start Toward Getting Fit

When Shopping for a Health Club

1. What types of services and facilities are you interested in (aerobics classes, court facilities,

pool, track, exercise machines, personal trainers)? Are the facilities well maintained?

2. If you know a member, get his or her honest, insider's opinion.

3. Is the club in a convenient location?

4. Are the operating hours compatible with your lifestyle?

5. Visit during the time of day you would use the club. Is it overcrowded? Could you use the equipment you want to work out on?

6. Is the fitness staff well qualified? Do they have degrees or certifications in a health/fitness related field? Are they trained in CPR and first aid?

7. Is the club reputable? How long has it been around? Do the management and personnel change often?

8. Do you have to sign a membership contract? Make sure you understand the commitment you're making and that all of your questions are answered before signing. Get a copy of your agreement.

9. What membership dues payment options do you have? Who are you actually paying?

10. What is their cancellation policy?

11. Try before you buy! Do they offer a free trial membership?

When Looking for a Personal Trainer

12. Is the trainer certified through a reputable organization such as:

    A.C.E. (American Council on Exercise)

    A.C.S.M. (American College of Sports Medicine)

13. Is the trainer certified in CPR and first aid?

14. Does the trainer have his or her own equipment or access to equipment? Can he or she come to your club to train you?

15. Can the trainer supply you with references from current and past clients?

When Looking into Exercise Classes

16. Are you familiar with the type of class (step, low impact)? If not, is the instructor willing to spend some time before class to give you a few pointers?

17. Is the format of the class safe? Does it include a warm-up, stretching, cardiovascular portion and a cool-down?

18. Is the class area big enough to safely accommodate the number of participants?

19. Does the floor of the aerobics area provide shock absorption to prevent injury? Athletic shoes specifically designed for and labeled as aerobic are the best choice for safety.

20. Are the instructors well qualified? Do they have instructor certifications through a reputable organization?

21. Try a class to see how you like the format and instructor.

When Purchasing Home Exercise Equipment

22. Is the store knowledgeable and reputable in the fitness and exercise equipment industry?

23. Can the sales staff explain how each piece of equipment works and what the differences are between models within a line or from different manufacturers?

24. Can you try the equipment in the store?

25. What are the store policies regarding trial use of equipment at home or returns?

26. Are electrical and outlet requirements for electrically run equipment (such as a treadmill) fully explained before purchasing?

27. Are product guarantees or warranties explained?

28. Does the store deliver and set up the equipment?

29. Who would repair equipment, the store itself? Or do they send it out? Who pays for pick-up and delivery? How long would you have to wait for repairs? Are repair charges explained?

When Purchasing Exercise/Fitness Tapes

30. Is the workout appropriate for your fitness level?

31. Does the workout require any equipment such as a step or toning apparatus?

32. Do you have enough room to do routines safely?

33. Is your floor surface carpeted to provide any shock absorption?

34. Is the instructor knowledgeable and reputable in the health and fitness industry? If not, do they credit someone with providing them training for the workout (for example, celebrity tapes)?

35. As your fitness level increases, can you vary the routine to keep it challenging? Does the instructor offer tips on varying the workout to suit different levels of fitness?

36. Video rental stores and libraries now offer exercise tapes; check one out and try it at home first.

The Activity Pyramid

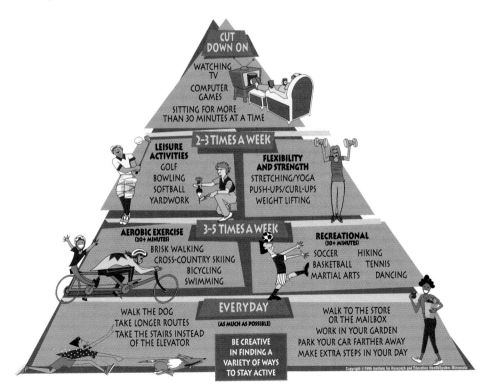

Source: Institute for Research and Education HealthSystem Minnesota. Copyright © 1997 by Institute for Research and Education. Reprinted by permission.

Calories Burned in Various Physical Activities

Activity	Calories per Minute	Activity	Calories per Minute
Aerobics		Gymnastics	
Low-intensity	3–4	balancing	3
High-intensity	8–10	abdominal	3
Archery	5	trunk bending	4
Badminton		hopping	7
recreation	5	Handball	10
competition	10	Hiking	
Baseball (except pitcher)	5	downhill, 5–10 percent grade (2.5 mph)	4
Basketball		downhill, 15–20 percent grade (2.5 mph)	4
half court	6	road/field (3.5 mph)	6–7
fastbreak	9	snow, soft–hard (2.5–3.5 mph)	10–20
Bowling (while active)	7	uphill, 5–15 percent grade (3.5 mph)	8–16
Calisthenics	6–8	Hill climbing (100 feet/hour)	8
Canoeing (2.5–4.0 mph)	3–7	Hockey	12–15
Carpentry	4	Horseback riding	
Cleaning windows	4	trot	5
Clerical work	1–2	walk	2
Cycling		Horseshoes	4
fast (12 mph)	8–10	Ironing clothes	4
slow (6 mph)	4–5	Jogging alternated with walking,	
10-speed bicycle (5–15 mph)	4–12	5 miles each	10
Dancing (moderate to vigorous)	4–8	Judo and karate	13
Dishwashing	1	Knitting or crocheting	0.5–0.8
Dressing	3	Making beds	3
Driving car	3	Meal preparation	3
Driving motorcycle	3	Mopping floors	5
Dusting	3	Mountain climbing	10
Eating	3	Mowing lawn	6
Farming chores		Piano playing	2
haying	7	Plastering walls	4
planting	5	Pool or billiards	2
Football (while active)	13	Racquetball	
Gardening		recreation	8
digging	9	competition	12
weeding	6	Reclining (watching TV)	2
		Roller blading/skating	
		(moderate to vigorous)	5–15

Activity	Calories per Minute	Activity	Calories per Minute
Rowing		Sweeping with:	
pleasure	5	broom	2
vigorous	15	vacuum cleaner	3
Running		Swimming	
8-minute mile (7.5 mph)	11	pleasure	6
6-minute mile (10 mph)	20	backstroke, breaststroke, crawl	
5-minute mile (12 mph)	25	(25–50 yards/minute)	6–13
Sawing		butterfly (50 yards/minute)	14
chain saw	6.2	Table tennis	5
crosscut saw	8–11	Talking	1
Sewing (hand or machine)	1	Tennis	
Shining shoes	3	recreation	7
Shoveling (depends on weight of load,		competition	11
rate of work, height of lift)	5–11	Tree felling (ax)	8–13
Showering	3	Truck and auto repair	4
Singing in loud voice	1	Typing (rapidly)	1
Sitting quietly	1	Volleyball	
Skipping rope	10–15	recreation	4
Skiing (snow)		competition	8
moderate to steep	8–12	Walking	
downhill racing	17	5-minute mile (12 mph)	25
cross-country (3.8 mph)	11–20	4 mph	6–7
Sleeping	1	3 mph	4–5
Snowshoeing (2.5 mph)	10	downstairs	4
Soccer	9	upstairs	8–10
Stair climber, light to moderate	8	Washing and dressing	3
Standing, light activity	3	Washing clothes	3
Standing, relaxed	1	Washing car	3
Step aerobics		Water skiing	8
4-inch step	5	Weight training	4
6-inch step	6	Wrestling	14
8-inch step	7	Writing	1

Source: General Mills, Inc.

Daily Exercise Tracker

Exercising three to five times per week for twenty to thirty minutes is recommended for overall health and fitness benefits. Weight loss will occur more quickly if exercise is increased to five times per week for forty-five to sixty minutes. Keep track of your daily exercise by referring to Calories Burned in Various Physical Activities.

Date	Activity	Time (in minutes)	Calories × per = Minute	Calories Burned	Before	After

Total Calories Burned = _____

Target Heart Rate

During your exercise session, pause and take your pulse to check you exercise intensity or training heart rate. You may choose one of two locations to take your pulse:

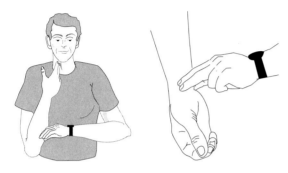

Your carotid artery (just to either side of the center of your neck)

Your radial artery (your wrist)

Apply light pressure with your fingers (don't use your thumb). Count how many beats you feel in a ten-second time period. Refer to the Target Heart Rate Chart below to see if you are working within your proper training range.

First, find your age range down the left side of the chart and move across to the number of beats you counted in ten seconds.

Now move up to the top of the chart to the percentage rates. These rates indicate that percentage of your maximum heart rate (which can be found by subtracting your age from 220). The numbers below these percentage rates indicate the number of beats (in a ten-second period) you would need to be working at to achieve that percentage rate or intensity level.

To receive the maximum benefit of your aerobic workout, do not exceed the 85 percent level. If you're just beginning an exercise program, aim for an intensity range of 60 percent. As your aerobic conditioning increases and you increase the intensity of your workouts, you will be more comfortable working closer to the 70 to 85 percent range.

Target Heart Rate Chart
10-Second Count

Age	60%	% A l l o w a b l e M a x i m u m 70%	75%	80%	85%
Under 20	21	25	26	28	30
20	20	23	25	27	28
25	20	23	24	26	28
30	19	22	24	25	27
35	19	22	23	25	26
40	18	21	23	24	26
45	18	21	22	23	25
50	17	20	21	23	24
55	17	19	21	22	23
60	16	19	20	21	22
65	16	18	19	21	22
70	15	18	19	20	21
75	15	17	18	19	21

Source: Stretching, Inc., P.O. Box 768, Palmer Lake, CO 80133.

The F.I.T. Principle

The F.I.T. Principle is an easy way for people to evaluate their workouts. It can be an answer to questions pertaining to frequency, intensity, and time or length of workouts.

If your goal is to achieve cardiovascular benefits and burn a significant number of calories, follow these guidelines:

F: Frequency
Exercise aerobically three to five times per week. This will help to achieve cardiovascular improvement as well as weight reduction.

I: Intensity
To maximize your training, you should be working at an intensity level of 60 to 80 percent of your maximum heart rate (see Target Heart Rate Chart, page 23). This is called your *target heart rate*. You may also chose to monitor your intensity through your level of *perceived exertion* (see Borg's Scale of Perceived Exertion on this page).

T: Time
To achieve cardiovascular benefits as well as sufficient caloric expenditure, exercise sessions should last between twenty and sixty minutes, excluding warm-up and cool-down time. Beginners may need to start at five or ten minutes and increase their time according to their comfort level. Ideally during this time, you should be working within your target heart rate zone.

Credit: Information from the American College of Sports Medicine Guidelines for Exercise Testing and Prescription (1995).

Perceived Exertion

Another means of monitoring exercise intensity is with the Borg's Rate of Perceived Exertion Scale (below). This scale is used to help determine a "comfort zone" while working out. You should be able to breathe both rhythmically and confortably while exercising to ensure a safe exercise level, especially if you are just beginning an exercise program.

Although the numbers on the scale correspond to a heart rate, this is a subjective test based on how you feel. Assign a numerical value between 6 and 20 that you would like to achieve for your exercise intensity, with 6 being very, very light and 20 being very, very difficult. A perceived exertion level of between 11 and 15 on the scale will approximately correspond to an intensity level of 60 percent (intensity range for a beginner exerciser) to 85 percent (maximum level for a good aerobic workout) of an individual's maximum heart rate.

Borg's Scale of Perceived Exertion

6	
7	Very, very light
8	
9	Very light
10	
11	Fairly light
12	
13	
14	
15	Hard
16	
17	Very hard
18	
19	Very, very hard
20	

Source: Guidelines for Exercise Testing and Prescription, *American College of Sports Medicine.*

Exercise "Cheaters"

Time is a precious commodity today. But making time, even in small amounts, to move your body will help and make you feel better about yourself. Some activities are listed below, but we're sure we haven't thought of everything! Add your own ingenious exercises.

- Take the stairs instead of the escalator or elevator.
- Do yard work.
- Park your car at the end of a row of spaces or farther from the entrance.
- Use idle time (airport layovers, medical appointments, waiting to be seated in a restaurant) to take a walk.
- Walk, bike or in-line skate to work rather than driving or busing.
- Schedule walk dates instead of lunch dates.
- Mow the lawn.
- Walk around the entire shopping center instead of just select stores.
- Wash the car by hand.
- Carry your own groceries.
- Walk the dog.
- Make more than one trip, such as carrying laundry, etc.
- Do housework to music.
- Avoid shortcuts.

Step 3: Go for the Goals

When thinking about goals, consider this motto: "Live one day at a time and count each and every one of your successes, you've earned them."

Goals can be short or long term. In fact, it's a good idea to have both types of goals, as that makes reaching them more realistic and manageable. Setting goals has a positive impact on motivation and attitude. As an example of motivation, think of training and competing to earn a spot on the U.S. Olympic Team. For each small goal reached along the way you feel proud and good about yourself, and this positive attitude helps you move forward.

Short-Term Goals: Examples of short-term goals might be:

- eating a piece of fruit instead of a doughnut during a break.
- walking during your lunch break instead of sitting in the cafeteria.
- using jelly or jam on your bagel instead of peanut butter or cream cheese.

Long-Term Goals: Examples of long-term goals might be:

- maintaining your healthy weight.
- establishing a regular exercise routine.
- maintaining a healthy eating pattern.

Setbacks: Don't put yourself down for setbacks; we all have them. If you ate six chocolate chip cookies yesterday, just forget about it and move on. A common mistake made after overeating is that people fast or skip meals; unfortunately, it only causes hunger and frustration. It's better for you just to follow your healthful eating plan starting with the next meal. For more ideas on "crisis management," refer to "Solutions for Problem Eating" on pages 138–139.

Rewards: You can reward yourself each time you reach a goal; just be sure the rewards are not food rewards. You might take a long, luxurious bubble bath or get a professional massage.

Comparison of Height and Weight

Before you determine your weight goal, record your body measurements on the Body Measurement Tracker on page 29. With good food choices and exercise, it will feel good to see the inches melt away.

To determine your weight goal, use the Metropolitan Life Insurance Table below or the Gerontology Research Center Table on the next page as a guide. Fill in the Weight goal and the "Alert" weight lines on the Weekly Weight Tracker on page 28.

Weigh in regularly once a week and at the same time of day. You can enjoy your progress and keep an alert for pounds creeping back. Remember to reward yourself each week you have lost weight. The reward doesn't have to be time-consuming or expensive, but rather something special for yourself, because you deserve it.

Metropolitan Life Insurance Table

Height	Men			Women		
	Small frame	Medium frame	Large frame	Small frame	Medium frame	Large frame
4'10"				102–111	109–121	118–131
4'11"				103–113	111–123	120–134
5'0"				104–115	113–126	122–137
5'1"				106–118	115–129	125–140
5'2"	128–134	131–141	138–150	108–121	118–132	128–143
5'3"	130–136	133–143	140–153	111–124	121–135	131–147
5'4"	132–138	135–145	142–156	114–127	124–138	134–151
5'5"	134–140	137–148	144–160	117–130	127–141	137–155
5'6"	136–142	139–151	146–164	120–133	130–144	140–159
5'7"	138–145	142–154	149–168	123–136	133–147	143–163
5'8"	140–148	145–157	152–172	126–139	136–150	146–167
5'9"	142–151	148–160	155–176	129–142	139–153	149–170
5'10"	144–154	151–163	158–180	132–145	142–156	152–173
5'11"	146–157	154–166	161–184	135–148	145–159	155–176
6'0"	149–160	157–170	164–188	138–151	148–162	158–179
6'1"	152–164	160–174	168–190			
6'2"	155–168	164–178	172–197			
6'3"	158–172	167–182	176–202			
6'4"	162–176	171–187	181–207			

All heights without shoes, weights in pounds without clothes. Weights at ages 25–59 based on lowest mortality. Weight in pounds according to frame (in indoor clothing weighing five pounds for men and three pounds for women; shoes with one-inch heels).

Source: Society of Actuaries and Association of Life Insurance Medical Directors of America.

Gerontology Research Center Table

Height	Age 20–29	Age 30–39	Age 40–49	Age 50–59	Age 60–69
4'10"	84–111	92–119	99–127	107–135	115–142
4'11"	87–115	95–123	103–131	111–139	119–147
5'0"	90–119	98–127	106–135	114–143	123–152
5'1"	93–123	101–131	110–140	118–148	127–157
5'2"	96–127	105–136	113–144	122–153	131–163
5'3"	99–131	108–140	117–149	126–158	135–168
5'4"	102–135	112–145	121–154	130–163	140–173
5'5"	106–140	115–149	125–159	134–168	144–179
5'6"	109–144	119–154	129–164	138–174	148–184
5'7"	112–148	122–159	133–169	143–179	153–190
5'8"	116–153	126–163	137–174	147–184	158–196
5'9"	119–157	130–168	141–179	151–190	162–201
5'10"	122–162	134–173	145–184	156–195	167–207
5'11"	126–167	137–178	149–190	160–201	172–213
6'0"	129–171	141–183	153–195	165–207	177–219
6'1"	133–176	145–188	157–200	169–213	182–235
6'2"	137–181	149–194	162–206	174–219	187–232
6'3"	141–186	153–199	166–212	179–225	192–238
6'4"	144–191	157–205	171–218	184–231	197–244

How to Approximate Your Frame Size

To determine your elbow breadth, extend your arm and bend the forearm upward at a 90-degree angle. Keep fingers straight and turn the inside of your wrist toward your body. If you have a caliper, use it to measure the space between the two prominent bones on *either side* of your elbow. Without a caliper, place thumb and index finger of your other hand on these two bones. Measure the space between your fingers against a ruler or tape measure. Compare it with these tables that list elbow measurements for *medium-framed* men and women. Measurements lower than those listed indicate you have a small frame. Higher measurements indicate a large frame.

Men		Women	
Height in 1" heels	**Elbow breadth**	**Height in 1" heels**	**Elbow breadth**
5'2"–5'3"	2 1/2"–2 7/8"	4'10"–4'11"	2 1/4"–2 1/2"
5'4"–5'7"	2 6/8"–2 7/8"	5'0"–5'3"	2 1/4"–2 1/2"
5'8"–5'11"	2 3/4"–3"	5'4"–5'7"	2 3/8"–2 5/8"
6'0"–6'3"	2 3/4"–3 1/8"	5'8"–5'11"	2 3/8"–2 5/8"
6'4"	2 7/8"–3 1/4"	6'0"	2 1/2"–2 3/4"

Weekly Weight Tracker

Starting date _____   **Weight goal** _____   **"Alert" weight** _____

Enter starting weight for Week 1 in the Weight column. Weigh in weekly, using the same scale and at the same time of day. Set an "alert" weight of five to seven pounds above your goal weight; reevaluate your eating and exercise habits when you reach your "alert" weight. If desired, record rewards each week weight is lost. Rewards should not be food related.

Week	Weight	Rewards
Week 1		
Week 2		
Week 3		
Week 4		
Week 5		
Week 6		
Week 7		
Week 8		
Week 9		
Week 10		
Week 11		
Week 12		
Week 13		
Week 14		
Week 15		
Week 16		
Week 17		
Week 18		
Week 19		
Week 20		
Week 21		
Week 22		

Body Measurement Tracker

Before you begin using Betty Crocker's 3-Step Guide, take your measurements and record them here. Take the measurements once each month.

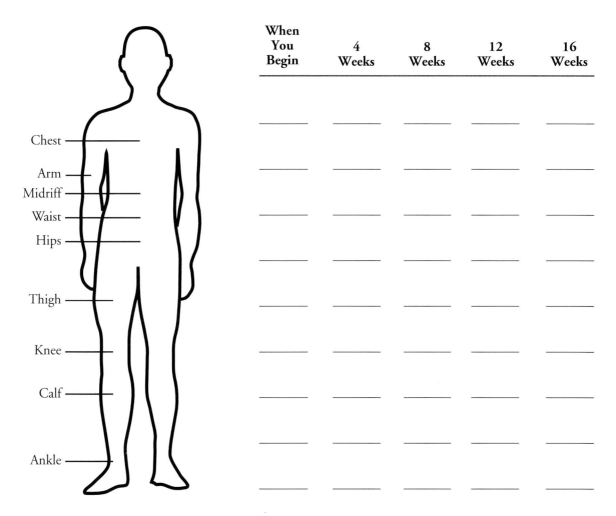

	When You Begin	4 Weeks	8 Weeks	12 Weeks	16 Weeks
Chest	_____	_____	_____	_____	_____
Arm / Midriff	_____	_____	_____	_____	_____
Waist	_____	_____	_____	_____	_____
Hips	_____	_____	_____	_____	_____
Thigh	_____	_____	_____	_____	_____
Knee	_____	_____	_____	_____	_____
Calf	_____	_____	_____	_____	_____
Ankle	_____	_____	_____	_____	_____
	_____	_____	_____	_____	_____

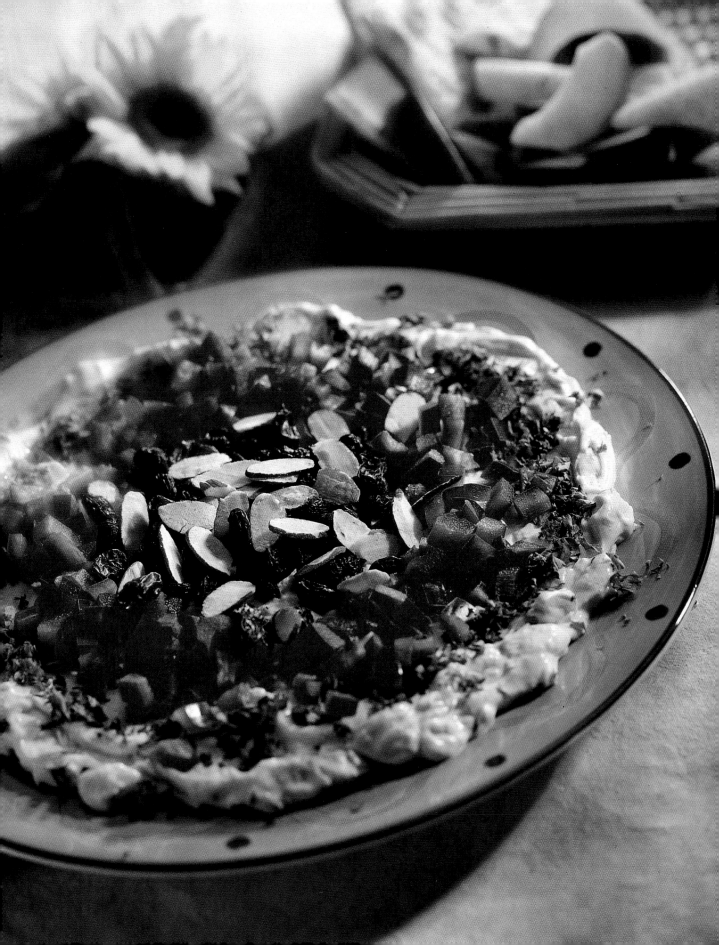

1
Appetizers and Snacks

Chicken Curry Spread
(page 33)

Almost Guacamole

PREP: 10 min; CHILL: 1 hr

ABOUT 2 CUPS DIP

1 can (15 ounces) asparagus cuts, drained

1 large tomato, seeded and chopped (1 cup)

1 medium onion, chopped (1/2 cup)

2 tablespoons finely chopped fresh cilantro

2 tablespoons reduced-fat mayonnaise or salad dressing

1 tablespoon lime juice

3 to 6 drops red pepper sauce

Dash of pepper

1 clove garlic, finely chopped

Baked tortilla chips, if desired

Place asparagus in blender or food processor. Cover and blend on medium speed until smooth.

Mix asparagus and remaining ingredients except tortilla chips. Cover and refrigerate at least 1 hour to blend flavors. Serve with tortilla chips.

1 Tablespoon:		% Daily Value:	
Calories	5	Vitamin A	0%
Calories from fat	0	Vitamin C	6%
Fat, g	0	Calcium	0%
Saturated, g	0	Iron	0%
Cholesterol, mg	0	**Diet Exchanges:**	
Sodium, mg	50	No exchanges	
Carbohydrate, g	1		
Dietary Fiber, g	0		
Protein, g	0		

Tangy Yogurt Dip

PREP: 2 min; CHILL: 1 hr

ABOUT 1 CUP DIP

1 cup plain fat-free yogurt

2 tablespoons chili sauce

1 to 2 teaspoons prepared horseradish

Assorted fresh vegetables, if desired

Mix all ingredients except vegetables. Cover and refrigerate at least 1 hour to blend flavors. Serve with vegetables.

1 Tablespoon:		% Daily Value:	
Calories	10	Vitamin A	0%
Calories from fat	0	Vitamin C	0%
Fat, g	0	Calcium	2%
Saturated, g	0	Iron	0%
Cholesterol, mg	0	**Diet Exchanges:**	
Sodium, mg	35	No exchanges	
Carbohydrate, g	2		
Dietary Fiber, g	0		
Protein, g	1		

Chicken Curry Spread

PREP: 10 min

4 CUPS SPREAD

For a more dramatic presentation, use a variety of colored bell peppers—green, red, yellow—whatever combination you choose. Another idea is to arrange bell peppers, raisins and almonds on the curry spread in concentric circles or stripes.

1 package (8 ounces) fat-free cream cheese, softened

1 cup fat-free sour cream

1 1/2 teaspoons curry powder

1/2 teaspoon salt

1/4 teaspoon ground ginger

1 cup finely chopped cooked chicken breast

1 medium bell pepper, chopped (1 cup)

1/3 cup raisins

1/4 cup sliced almonds, toasted

Chopped parsley, if desired

Apple and pear slices, if desired

Beat cream cheese, sour cream, curry powder, salt and ginger in medium bowl until smooth. Stir in chicken. Spread mixture on flat plate, about 9 to 10 inches in diameter. Sprinkle with bell pepper, raisins, almonds and parsley. Serve with apple and pear slices.

1 Tablespoon:		% Daily Value:	
Calories	10	Vitamin A	0%
Calories from fat	0	Vitamin C	2%
Fat, g	0	Calcium	0%
Saturated, g	0	Iron	0%
Cholesterol, mg	2	**Diet Exchanges:**	
Sodium, mg	45	No exchanges	
Carbohydrate, g	1		
Dietary Fiber, g	0		
Protein, g	1		

IS FAT-FREE ALWAYS BEST?

Fact: Fat-free and low-fat foods are low in calories.

False: Just because fat has been removed from food, doesn't necessarily mean the calories have been reduced. When food manufacturers remove fat, other components, usually carbohydrates, are added to improve the taste and texture of the reduced-fat food. Check the labels on these products to be sure you're not overindulging on these foods.

Fact: Fat-free and low-fat foods are always healthier than regular foods.

False: Foods with less fat often appear to be a better choice than their regular counterparts. However, read nutrition labels on packaged products to be sure. Often, when fat is removed, so is flavor. And to make up for the loss in flavor, extra calories, sugars and salt may be added to boost the taste.

Mushroom Pita Pizzas

PREP: 10 min; BAKE: 10 min

8 SERVINGS (4 PIECES OR 1/2 ROUND EACH)

2 pita breads (6 inches in diameter)

2 cups sliced mushrooms* (6 ounces)

1 small red onion, thinly sliced

1/4 cup chopped green bell pepper

2 tablespoons chopped fresh or 2 teaspoons dried basil leaves

1 cup finely shredded reduced-fat mozzarella cheese (4 ounces)

1 tablespoon grated fat-free Parmesan cheese

Heat oven to 425°. Split each pita bread around edge with knife to make 2 rounds. Place rounds, cut sides up, on ungreased cookie sheet. Top rounds with mushrooms, onion and bell pepper. Sprinkle with basil and cheeses. Bake 8 to 10 minutes or until cheese is melted. Cut each round into 8 wedges.

*1 can (4 ounces) mushroom stems and pieces, drained, can be substituted for the fresh mushrooms.

4 Pieces:		% Daily Value:	
Calories	80	Vitamin A	6%
Calories from fat	20	Vitamin C	2%
Fat, g	2	Calcium	10%
Saturated, g	1	Iron	4%
Cholesterol, mg	0	Diet Exchanges:	
Sodium, mg	190	1 starch/bread	
Carbohydrate, g	14		
Dietary Fiber, g	1		
Protein, g	3		

Italian Salsa

PREP: 15 min; CHILL: 1 hr

2 3/4 CUPS SALSA

For a change of pace, serve this fresh Italian version of salsa with toasted French or Italian bread slices.

2 large tomatoes, chopped (2 cups)

1 small onion, chopped (1/4 cup)

1/3 cup finely chopped green bell pepper

1/3 cup chopped ripe olives

2 tablespoons red wine vinegar

1 tablespoon olive or vegetable oil

2 tablespoons chopped fresh basil leaves

2 cloves garlic, finely chopped

Mix all ingredients in nonmetal bowl. Cover and refrigerate at least 1 hour to blend flavors.

1/4 Cup:		% Daily Value:	
Calories	15	Vitamin A	2%
Calories from fat	10	Vitamin C	12%
Fat, g	1	Calcium	0%
Saturated, g	0	Iron	2%
Cholesterol, mg	0	Diet Exchanges:	
Sodium, mg	30	No exchanges	
Carbohydrate, g	2		
Dietary Fiber, g	0		
Protein, g	0		

Italian Salsa

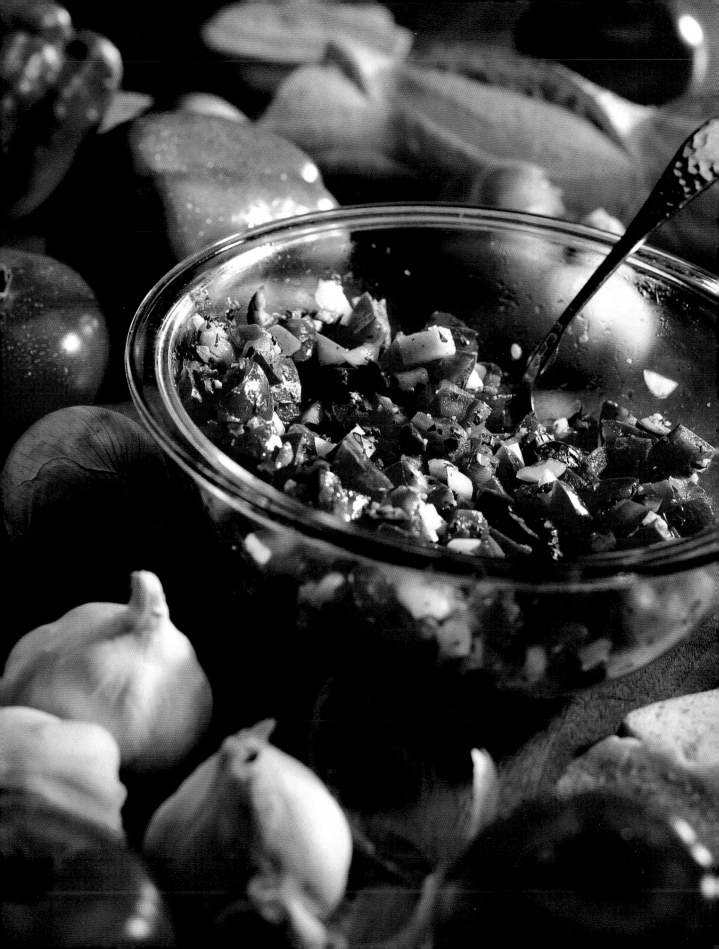

Cucumbers, Carrots and Smoked Salmon Crudités

PREP: 15 min

24 APPETIZERS

Isn't it great to know that appetizers don't always have to be fat traps? And, by using carrot or cucumber slices instead of crackers, this healthful appetizer is even lower in fat and calories!

2 ounces salmon lox, finely chopped

1/2 cup fat-free soft cream cheese, softened

3/4 teaspoon chopped fresh or 1/4 teaspoon dried dill weed

2 large cucumbers or carrots, cut into 1/4-inch slices (24 slices)

Dill weed sprigs, if desired

Mix lox, cream cheese and chopped dill weed. Place lox mixture in decorating bag fitted with large star tip, and pipe 1 heaping teaspoonful onto each carrot slice; or spoon lox mixture onto each carrot slice. Garnish each with dill weed sprig.

1 Appetizer:		% Daily Value:	
Calories	10	Vitamin A	14%
Calories from fat	0	Vitamin C	2%
Fat, g	0	Calcium	0%
Saturated, g	0	Iron	0%
Cholesterol, mg	0	**Diet Exchanges:**	
Sodium, mg	55	No exchanges	
Carbohydrate, g	1		
Dietary Fiber, g	0		
Protein, g	1		

Cucumbers, Carrots and Smoked Salmon Crudités

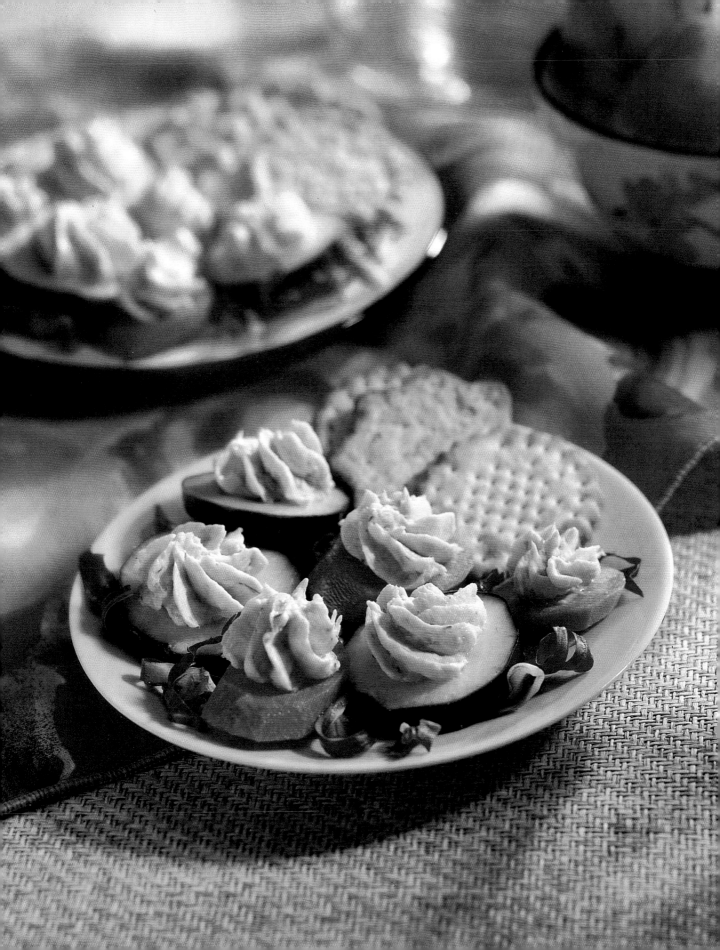

Curried Meatballs with Chutney Sauce

PREP: 10 min; CHILL: 1 hr; BAKE: 15 min

4 DOZEN APPETIZERS

Chutney Sauce (below)

1 pound ground turkey breast

1/2 cup crushed cracker crumbs

1/3 cup evaporated skimmed milk

1 1/2 to 2 teaspoons curry powder

1/4 teaspoon salt

**2 medium green onions, finely chopped
(2 tablespoons)**

Prepare Chutney Sauce.

Heat oven to 400°. Mix remaining ingredients. Shape mixture into forty-eight 1-inch meatballs. Place in ungreased rectangular pan, 13 × 9 × 2 inches. Bake uncovered 10 to 15 minutes or until no longer pink in center and light brown on outside. Serve hot with Chutney Sauce.

CHUTNEY SAUCE

1/2 cup plain fat-free yogurt

**1 tablespoon finely chopped chutney or
peach preserves**

1/4 teaspoon curry powder

Mix all ingredients. Cover and refrigerate at least 1 hour to blend flavors.

1 Appetizer:		% Daily Value:	
Calories	20	Vitamin A	0%
Calories from fat	10	Vitamin C	0%
Fat, g	1	Calcium	0%
Saturated, g	0	Iron	0%
Cholesterol, mg	5	**Diet Exchanges:**	
Sodium, mg	30	No exchanges	
Carbohydrate, g	1		
Dietary Fiber, g	0		
Protein, g	2		

Peppery Mini-Bites

PREP: 10 min; COOK: 5 min; BAKE: 10 min

22 APPETIZERS

**1 small red or green bell pepper, chopped
(1/2 cup)**

**4 medium green onions, finely chopped
(1/4 cup)**

**1 cup fat-free cholesterol-free egg product or
2 eggs plus 3 egg whites**

**1/2 cup shredded reduced-fat Cheddar
cheese (2 ounces)**

1 teaspoon chili powder

1/2 teaspoon ground cumin

1/8 teaspoon ground red pepper (cayenne)

**1 can (4 ounces) chopped green chilies, well
drained**

Heat oven to 425°. Spray 10-inch nonstick skillet with nonstick cooking spray; heat over medium-high heat. Cook bell pepper and onions in skillet about 5 minutes, stirring occasionally, until onions are tender.

Spray small muffin cups, 1 3/4 × 1 inch, with nonstick cooking spray. Mix bell pepper mixture and remaining ingredients. Spoon 1 tablespoon mixture into each muffin cup. Bake 8 to 10 minutes or until centers are set. Cool 1 minute. Loosen edges with knife and remove from pan. Serve immediately.

1 Appetizer:		% Daily Value:	
Calories	10	Vitamin A	2%
Calories from fat	0	Vitamin C	6%
Fat, g	0	Calcium	2%
Saturated, g	0	Iron	2%
Cholesterol, mg	2	**Diet Exchanges:**	
Sodium, mg	75	No exchanges	
Carbohydrate, g	1		
Dietary Fiber, g	0		
Protein, g	2		

Phyllo Egg Rolls

PREP: 30 min; BAKE: 20 min

18 EGG ROLLS

These clever egg rolls are made without all the mess—and calories—of deep-frying.

1 pound ground turkey breast

4 cups coleslaw mix

3 tablespoons reduced-sodium soy sauce

1 teaspoon grated gingerroot

1/2 teaspoon five-spice powder

1 small onion, chopped (1/4 cup)

2 cloves garlic, finely chopped

18 frozen (thawed) phyllo sheets
    (16 × 12 inches)

Heat oven to 350°. Cook turkey in 10-inch skillet over medium-high heat, stirring occasionally, until no longer pink; drain. Stir in remaining ingredients except phyllo. Cook 2 to 3 minutes, stirring occasionally, until coleslaw mix is wilted; remove from heat.

Unroll phyllo sheets; cover sheets with waxed paper, then with damp towel to prevent them from drying out. Place 1 phyllo sheet on cutting board; spray with nonstick cooking spray. Repeat with 2 more phyllo sheets to make stack of 3 sheets. Cut stack of phyllo sheets crosswise into thirds to make 3 rectangles, about 12 × 5 inches.

Place 1/4 cup turkey mixture on short end of each rectangle; roll up, folding in edges of phyllo. Place roll, seam side down, on cookie sheet. Repeat with remaining phyllo and turkey mixture. Spray rolls with nonstick cooking spray. Bake 15 to 20 minutes or until light golden brown. Serve warm.

1 Egg Roll:		% Daily Value:	
Calories	95	Vitamin A	0%
Calories from fat	10	Vitamin C	4%
Fat, g	1	Calcium	2%
Saturated, g	0	Iron	6%
Cholesterol, mg	15	**Diet Exchanges:**	
Sodium, mg	190	1 starch/bread	
Carbohydrate, g	15		
Dietary Fiber, g	1		
Protein, g	8		

Fact Versus Fiction: Diet Claims

Q: Can eating certain foods such as grapefruit, or certain combinations of food, burn fat?

A: There is no food that will cause fat to be burned away. Eat sensibly, exercise regularly and you will lose fat.

Q: Can eating certain foods, such as celery, use up calories in the body?

A: There are some foods that have very few calories, but none will actually burn up calories by themselves, no matter how hard we chew!

Q: If I starve myself for a week, could I lose ten or more pounds?

A: If no food is eaten, yet normal activities remain the same, about two to three pounds a week can be lost. Under starvation conditions, the body must break down its own protein to maintain enough energy to function and protein by-products require an increase in water loss for excretion. Therefore, a very low calorie diet may cause *temporary* weight loss, which only amounts to water loss. The weight will be regained as soon as a more normal diet begins. It is extremely difficult to balance the necessary vitamins and minerals in a diet with less than 1,000 calories and almost impossible to do so in a diet providing less than 800 calories each day. Experts recommend not eating less than 1,200 calories per day.

Q: Do liquid diet supplements increase weight loss?

A: Liquid food supplements can be *temporarily* helpful in keeping calorie intake lower. If using this type of product, it is very important to maintain a balanced diet by eating at least one or two meals of "regular" food each day the supplement is used. Because the use of these products is short term, you will eventually have to return to the normal food world and it is important to learn to choose, prepare and eat good food choices. A word of caution about very low calorie liquid supplements: Because of the large amounts of water lost with these diets, when normal eating is resumed, the body compensates by retaining massive amounts of fluid, which can dilute the body's potassium and cause abnormal heart rhythms.

Q: Are natural foods are better for you?

A: *Natural* usually means that a food is taken directly from the food source, with no processing. It also refers to foods that have acquired a "healthy" label. Not only can the term *natural* be misinformation, but some foods that are considered natural can actually be less healthful. For example, raw peanuts contain toxic substances that are destroyed during roasting or cooking at high temperatures. The more important question is what kind of processing is involved (such as deep-fat frying) and what the breakdown of ingredients is in terms of fat, protein and carbohydrates. Some "natural" foods, such as coconut oil and some herbal teas, can cause specific increased health risks, including coronary artery disease, liver damage or severe allergies.

Q: Are diet pills safe?

A: Diet pills act by stimulating the "feeding center" in the brain to reduce the feeling of hunger. Unfortunately, the same stimulants act on other parts of the nervous system, typically causing insomnia, agitation and tremor at the doses required for weight reduction. Moreover, many of these stimulants carry the potential for addiction and abuse. Unfortunately, all of the existing medications are effective only when being maintained; the weight is regained upon stopping the medication. It is better to make lifelong changes to healthful eating habits and to exercise regularly.

Gorgonzola and Caramelized Onion Appetizer

PREP: 10 min; COOK: 25 min; BROIL: 5 min

4 SERVINGS

For easy last-minute assembly, the onions can be prepared and refrigerated up to 48 hours ahead of time.

2 tablespoons reduced-calorie spread

2 medium onions, sliced and separated into rings

1 tablespoon packed brown sugar

1/2 teaspoon balsamic or red wine vinegar

8 slices baguette, 1/2 inch thick

2 tablespoons crumbled Gorgonzola cheese

Melt spread in 10-inch skillet over medium heat. Cook onions, brown sugar and vinegar in spread about 25 minutes, stirring frequently, until onions are golden brown.

Set oven control to broil. Place baguette slices on cookie sheet. Broil with tops 2 to 3 inches from heat 1 to 2 minutes or until lightly toasted. Spoon caramelized onions evenly onto each slice. Sprinkle with cheese. Broil about 1 minute or until cheese is melted.

1 Serving:		% Daily Value:	
Calories	145	Vitamin A	8%
Calories from fat	45	Vitamin C	2%
Fat, g	5	Calcium	6%
Saturated, g	2	Iron	6%
Cholesterol, mg	5	**Diet Exchanges:**	
Sodium, mg	310	1 1/2 starch/bread	
Carbohydrate, g	23	1 fat	
Dietary Fiber, g	2		
Protein, g	4		

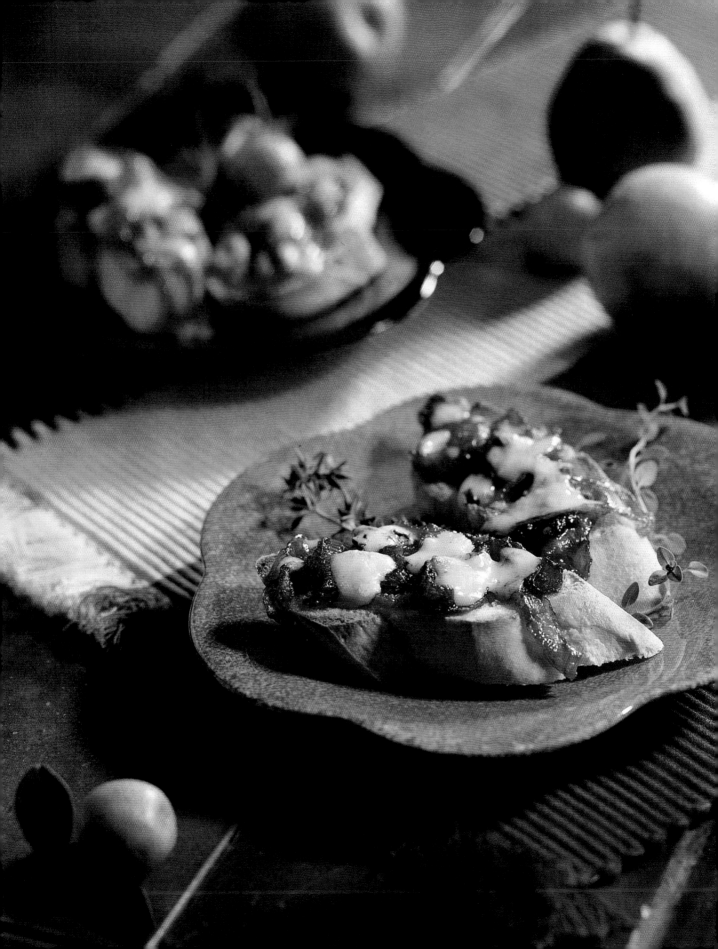

Black Bean–Corn Wonton Cups

PREP: 25 min; BAKE: 10 min

36 APPETIZERS

This recipe is great when you need appetizers that can be prepared ahead of time. Just bake the wonton cups ahead, and mix up the filling. Fill and garnish the wonton cups right before serving.

36 wonton skins

2/3 cup thick-and-chunky salsa

1/4 cup chopped fresh cilantro

1/2 teaspoon ground cumin

1/2 teaspoon chili powder

1 can (15 1/4 ounces) whole kernel corn, drained

1 can (15 ounces) black beans, rinsed and drained

1/4 cup plus 2 tablespoons fat-free sour cream

Cilantro sprigs, if desired

Heat oven to 350°. Gently fit 1 wonton skin into each of 36 small muffin cups, 1 3/4 × 1 inch. Bake 8 to 10 minutes or until light golden brown. Remove from pan; cool on wire racks.

Mix remaining ingredients except sour cream and cilantro sprigs. Just before serving, spoon bean mixture into wonton cups. Top each with 1/2 teaspoon sour cream. Garnish each with cilantro sprig.

1 Appetizer:		% Daily Value:	
Calories	50	Vitamin A	0%
Calories from fat	0	Vitamin C	0%
Fat, g	0	Calcium	2%
Saturated, g	0	Iron	4%
Cholesterol, mg	0	**Diet Exchanges:**	
Sodium, mg	120	2 vegetable	
Carbohydrate, g	11		
Dietary Fiber, g	1		
Protein, g	2		

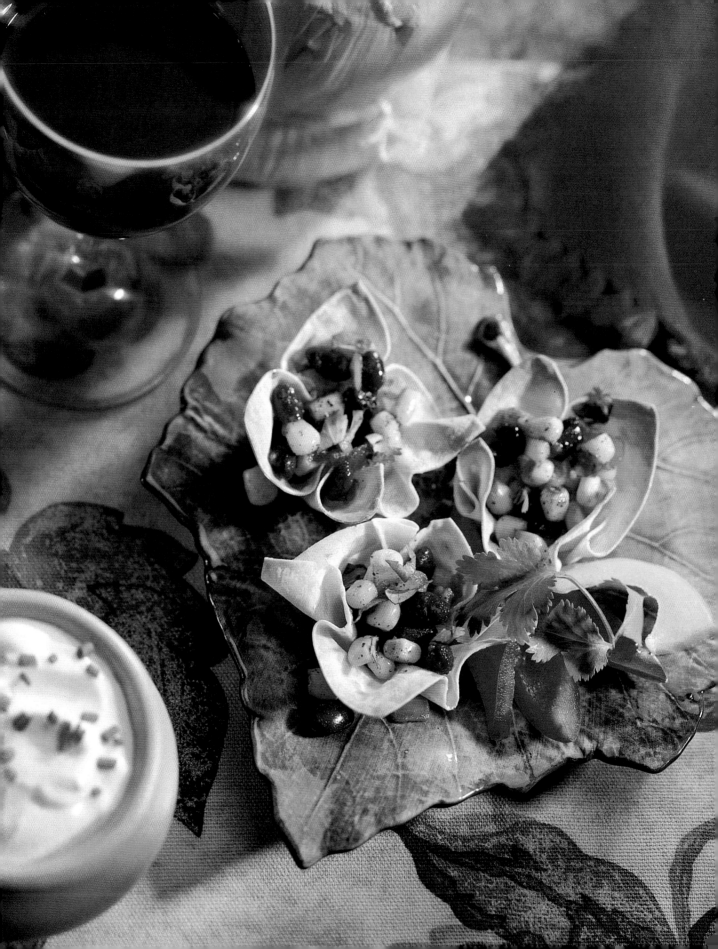

Savory Popcorn Mix

PREP: 10 min; BAKE: 30 min

ABOUT **9** CUPS SNACK

6 cups hot-air-popped popcorn

2 cups fat-free pretzel sticks

2 cups tiny fish-shaped crackers

2 tablespoons margarine, melted

1/2 teaspoon garlic powder

1/2 teaspoon onion powder

1/2 teaspoon dried basil leaves

1/2 teaspoon dried oregano leaves

1/8 to 1/4 teaspoon red pepper sauce

Heat oven to 300°. Mix popcorn, pretzel sticks and crackers in rectangular pan, 13 × 9 × 2 inches. Mix remaining ingredients. Drizzle over popcorn mixture; toss until evenly coated. Bake about 30 minutes, stirring every 10 minutes, until toasted. Serve warm. Store any leftover snack in tightly covered container.

1 Cup:		% Daily Value:	
Calories	130	Vitamin A	4%
Calories from fat	55	Vitamin C	0%
Fat, g	6	Calcium	0%
Saturated, g	2	Iron	4%
Cholesterol, mg	0	**Diet Exchanges:**	
Sodium, mg	290	1 starch/bread	
Carbohydrate, g	18	1 fat	
Dietary Fiber, g	1		
Protein, g	2		

Southwestern Popcorn Snack

PREP: 10 min

ABOUT **8** CUPS SNACK

6 cups hot-air-popped popcorn

2 cups Cheerios cereal

2 tablespoons margarine

1/2 teaspoon chili powder

1/4 teaspoon ground cumin

1/4 teaspoon garlic powder

2 tablespoons grated fat-free Parmesan cheese

Mix popcorn and cereal in large bowl. Heat margarine, chili powder, cumin and garlic powder until margarine is melted. Drizzle over popcorn mixture; toss until evenly coated. Immediately sprinkle with cheese; toss until evenly coated. Serve warm. Store any leftover snack in tightly covered container.

1 Cup:		% Daily Value:	
Calories	75	Vitamin A	12%
Calories from fat	35	Vitamin C	2%
Fat, g	4	Calcium	2%
Saturated, g	1	Iron	10%
Cholesterol, mg	2	**Diet Exchanges:**	
Sodium, mg	120	1/2 starch/bread	
Carbohydrate, g	9	1 fat	
Dietary Fiber, g	1		
Protein, g	2		

MUNCHIE ATTACK RESCUE

When you get an attack of the munchies, reach for one of the twenty ideas listed below—they are all are under 100 calories!

1. 100 thin (2 1/4-inch) fat-free pretzel sticks
2. 25 fresh or frozen grapes
3. 10 animal crackers
4. 8 baked tortilla chips with 1/4 cup salsa
5. 3 cups 94 percent fat-free microwave popcorn with 1 tablespoon fat-free grated Parmesan cheese
6. Three 2 1/2-inch graham cracker squares
7. 3 whole medium carrots
8. 3 small plums
9. 2 cups raw broccoli or cauliflower flowerets
10. 2 medium tangerines
11. 1 minibagel with 1 tablespoon reduced-fat or fat-free cream cheese
12. 1 frozen fudge bar
13. 1 100 percent fruit frozen juice bar
14. 1 medium banana
15. 1 cup sugar-free hot cocoa with 2 large marshmallows
16. 1 ounce raisins or dried berries (cranberries, cherries, blueberries)
17. 1/2 cup chocolate nonfat frozen yogurt with 1 tablespoon fresh raspberries
18. 1/2 cup lemon nonfat yogurt mixed with 1/2 cup fresh blueberries
19. 1/2 cup vanilla instant sugar-free fat-free pudding with 1 tablespoon light whipped topping
20. 1/4 cantaloupe topped with 1/2 cup nonfat vanilla yogurt

Spicy Carrots and Jicama

PREP: 15 min; CHILL: 2 hr

ABOUT **40** SERVINGS

1/4 cup lemon juice

2 teaspoons vegetable oil

1/2 teaspoon garlic powder

1/2 teaspoon chili powder

1/8 to 1/4 teaspoon ground red pepper (cayenne)

4 medium carrots (about 1/2 pound)

1/2 pound jicama, peeled

Shake all ingredients except carrots and jicama in tightly covered container. Cut carrots lengthwise into fourths; cut each fourth crosswise in half. Cut jicama into 3 × 1/4 × 1/4-inch strips.

Place carrots and jicama in nonmetal bowl or heavy-duty resealable plastic bag. Pour lemon juice mixture over vegetables; toss well to coat. Cover bowl or seal bag and refrigerate at least 2 hours to blend flavors, stirring occasionally. Drain before serving.

1 Serving (1/4 cup):		% Daily Value:	
Calories	10	Vitamin A	12%
Calories from fat	0	Vitamin C	0%
Fat, g	0	Calcium	0%
Saturated, g	0	Iron	0%
Cholesterol, mg	0	**Diet Exchanges:**	
Sodium, mg	0	No exchanges	
Carbohydrate, g	2		
Dietary Fiber, g	0		
Protein, g	0		

Frosty Mocha Cappuccino

PREP: **5 min**

4 SERVINGS

Instant coffee can easily be substituted for the fresh brewed, so you can make this refreshing drink whenever you like.

1 cup very strong coffee, cooled

2 cups vanilla fat-free ice cream

2 tablespoons chocolate-flavored syrup

Place all ingredients in blender or food processor. Cover and blend on high speed until smooth.

1 Serving:		% Daily Value:	
Calories	120	Vitamin A	8%
Calories from fat	0	Vitamin C	0%
Fat, g	0	Calcium	8%
Saturated, g	0	Iron	0%
Cholesterol, mg	0	**Diet Exchanges:**	
Sodium, mg	75	1 fruit	
Carbohydrate, g	26	1/2 skim milk	
Dietary Fiber, g	0		
Protein, g	4		

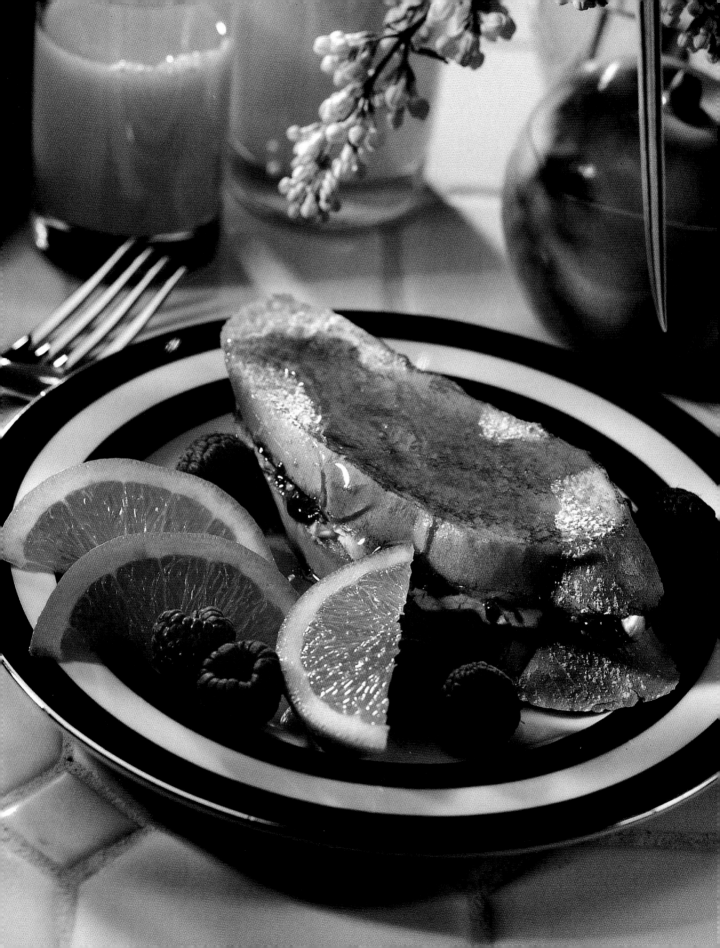

2

Breakfasts to Keep You Going

Stuffed French Toast
(page 58)

CHOLESTEROL MYTHS

Fact: Margarine, vegetable oil and peanut butter contain a lot of cholesterol.

False: These foods from vegetable sources don't provide cholesterol; however, they do provide a concentrated source of fat and calories. Only animal foods contain cholesterol.

Fact: Chicken and fish are cholesterol free.

False: Contrary to popular belief, chicken and fish do contain cholesterol. These foods supply less fat and saturated fat in general than do red meats such as beef and pork.

Fact: Foods low in cholesterol are low in fat too.

False: Whether or not a food contains cholesterol doesn't have any bearing on the amount of fat that's present in the food. Cholesterol is only found in foods of animal origin: meats, fish, poultry, some seafood and dairy products. But fat is found in both plant and animal foods.

Herbed Eggs with Salsa

PREP: 8 min; BAKE: 40 min; STAND: 5 min

6 SERVINGS

1 medium onion, chopped (1/2 cup)

1/2 cup shredded reduced-fat mozzarella cheese (2 ounces)

1 1/2 cups skim milk

1 cup fat-free cholesterol-free egg product or 2 eggs plus 3 egg whites

1/3 cup all-purpose flour

1 teaspoon Italian seasoning

1/4 teaspoon salt

3/4 cup salsa

Heat oven to 350°. Spray pie plate, 9×1 1/4 inches, with nonstick cooking spray. Sprinkle onion and cheese in pie plate. Place remaining ingredients except salsa in blender. Cover and blend on medium-high speed about 30 seconds or until smooth. Pour into pie plate.

Bake about 40 minutes or until knife inserted in center comes out clean. Let stand 5 minutes before serving. Serve with salsa.

1 Serving:		% Daily Value:	
Calories	90	Vitamin A	8%
Calories from fat	10	Vitamin C	6%
Fat, g	1	Calcium	18%
Saturated, g	0	Iron	4%
Cholesterol, mg	5	**Diet Exchanges:**	
Sodium, mg	320	1/2 starch/bread	
Carbohydrate, g	12	1/2 skim milk	
Dietary Fiber, g	1		
Protein, g	9		

Vegetable-Egg Fajitas

PREP: 15 min; COOK: 8 min

4 SERVINGS

The satisfying flavor of fajitas is not just for dinner anymore—try these fajitas to jazz up your morning.

1 1/2 cups fat-free cholesterol-free egg product

1/3 cup skim milk

1 tablespoon fajita seasoning mix (from 1.27-ounce envelope)

1 tablespoon vegetable oil

1 medium bell pepper, cut into 1/4-inch strips

1 medium onion, sliced and separated into rings

4 fat-free flour tortillas (6 to 8 inches in diameter)

1/2 cup salsa

Mix egg product, milk and fajita seasoning with fork; set aside. Heat oil in 12-inch nonstick skillet over medium-high heat. Cook bell pepper and onion in oil 2 to 3 minutes, stirring occasionally, until vegetables are tender.

Pour egg mixture into skillet. As mixture begins to set at bottom and side, gently lift cooked portions with spatula so that thin, uncooked portion can flow to bottom. Avoid constant stirring. Cook 3 to 4 minutes or until eggs are thickened throughout but still moist.

Spoon one-fourth of the egg mixture onto center of each tortilla. Fold one end of tortilla up about 1 inch over mixture; fold right and left sides over folded end, overlapping. Fold remaining end down. Serve each fajita topped with 2 tablespoons salsa.

1 Serving:		% Daily Value:	
Calories	225	Vitamin A	16%
Calories from fat	35	Vitamin C	22%
Fat, g	4	Calcium	10%
Saturated, g	1	Iron	20%
Cholesterol, mg	0	**Diet Exchanges:**	
Sodium, mg	930	2 starch/bread	
Carbohydrate, g	38	1 lean meat	
Dietary Fiber, g	4	1 vegetable	
Protein, g	13		

Lemon Muesli

PREP: 5 min

2 SERVINGS

Swiss nutritionist Dr. Bircher-Benner developed muesli as a health food near the end of the nineteenth century.

1/2 cup lemon fat-free yogurt

1/2 cup skim milk

1 tablespoon packed brown sugar

1 cup old-fashioned oats

2 tablespoons raisins or chopped dried fruit

1/2 medium banana, chopped

Mix yogurt, milk and brown sugar in medium bowl. Stir in oats and raisins. Spoon into 2 individual serving bowls. Top with banana before serving.

1 Serving:		% Daily Value:	
Calories	285	Vitamin A	10%
Calories from fat	25	Vitamin C	6%
Fat, g	3	Calcium	18%
Saturated, g	1	Iron	14%
Cholesterol, mg	2	**Diet Exchanges:**	
Sodium, mg	65	2 starch/bread	
Carbohydrate, g	59	1 1/2 fruit	
Dietary Fiber, g	5	1/2 skim milk	
Protein, g	11		

Wild Rice Frittata

PREP: 10 min; COOK: 20; STAND: 5

6 SERVINGS

1 tablespoon reduced-calorie spread

1 small green bell pepper, chopped (1/2 cup)

1 small red bell pepper, chopped (1/2 cup)

1 medium onion, chopped (1/2 cup)

1 1/2 cups fat-free cholesterol-free egg product

1/4 cup skim milk

1 cup cooked wild rice

1 cup shredded reduced-fat Swiss cheese (4 ounces)

Melt spread in 10-inch nonstick skillet over medium heat. Cook bell peppers and onion in spread, stirring frequently, until vegetables are crisp-tender.

Mix egg product, milk, wild rice and 1/2 cup of the cheese; pour over vegetables. Reduce heat to low. Cover and cook 15 to 20 minutes or until eggs are set; remove from heat. Sprinkle with remaining cheese. Cover and let stand about 5 minutes or until cheese is melted. Cut into wedges. Serve immediately.

1 Serving:		% Daily Value:	
Calories	125	Vitamin A	12%
Calories from fat	35	Vitamin C	18%
Fat, g	4	Calcium	26%
Saturated, g	2	Iron	8%
Cholesterol, mg	5	**Diet Exchanges:**	
Sodium, mg	130	1 lean meat	
Carbohydrate, g	11	1 vegetable	
Dietary Fiber, g	1	1/2 skim milk	
Protein, g	12		

Wild Rice Frittata

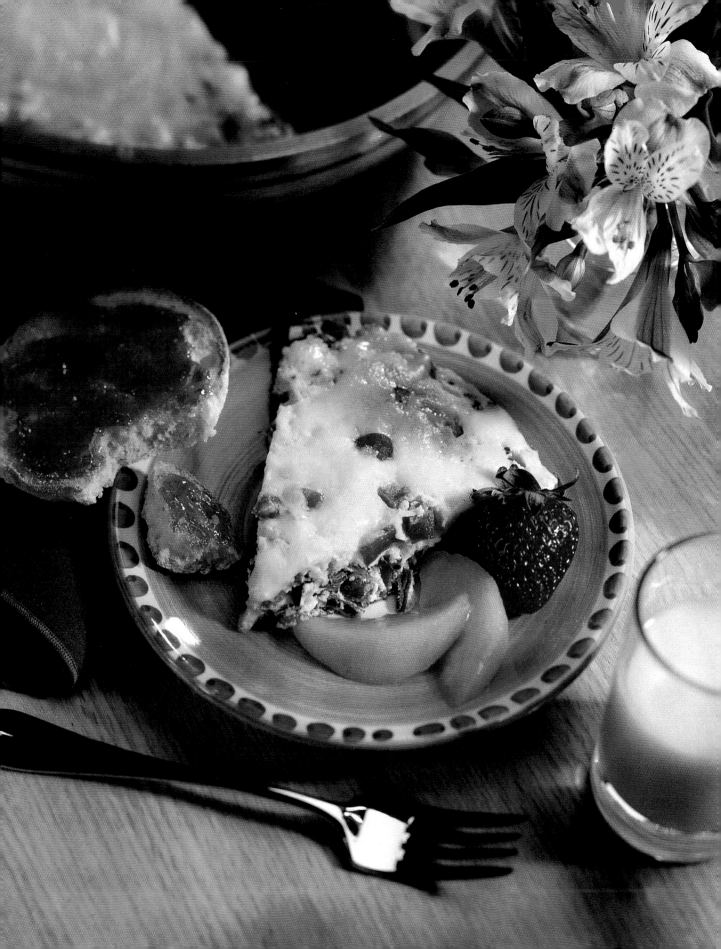

Mou Shu Pork Egg Pancakes

PREP: 20 min

4 SERVINGS

Mou Shu is a Chinese stir-fried dish containing shredded pork and various seasonings, and is typically served in a flour pancake. Try our egg pancake for a change of pace.

1/2 pound pork boneless butterfly chop

1 cup fat-free cholesterol-free egg product

1/4 cup skim milk

1/4 teaspoon salt

1/8 teaspoon pepper

3 cups broccoli slaw or coleslaw mix

1/4 cup plum sauce

2 teaspoons reduced-sodium soy sauce

Chinese mustard, if desired

Trim fat from pork. Cut pork into 1/4-inch strips. Mix egg product, milk, salt and pepper.

Spray 7- or 8-inch nonstick skillet with nonstick cooking spray; heat over medium heat. For each pancake, pour 2 to 3 tablespoons egg mixture into skillet, and quickly rotate skillet to coat bottom with egg, forming a thin layer. Cook about 2 minutes or until pancake is light golden brown around edge and center is almost set. Run wide spatula around edge to loosen; turn and cook other side until center is set. Repeat with remaining egg mixture, making 3 more pancakes. Stack pancakes between layers of waxed paper to prevent sticking; keep warm.

Spray 12-inch nonstick skillet with nonstick cooking spray; heat over medium-high heat. Cook pork in skillet 2 to 4 minutes, stirring occasionally, until no longer pink in center. Stir in remaining ingredients. Cook 4 to 5 minutes, stirring occasionally, until broccoli slaw is tender. Spoon 1/4 cup pork mixture down center of each pancake; roll up. Serve with Chinese mustard.

1 Serving:		% Daily Value:	
Calories	130	Vitamin A	4%
Calories from fat	35	Vitamin C	14%
Fat, g	4	Calcium	6%
Saturated, g	2	Iron	10%
Cholesterol, mg	30	**Diet Exchanges:**	
Sodium, mg	370	2 lean meat	
Carbohydrate, g	9	1/2 fruit	
Dietary Fiber, g	2		
Protein, g	17		

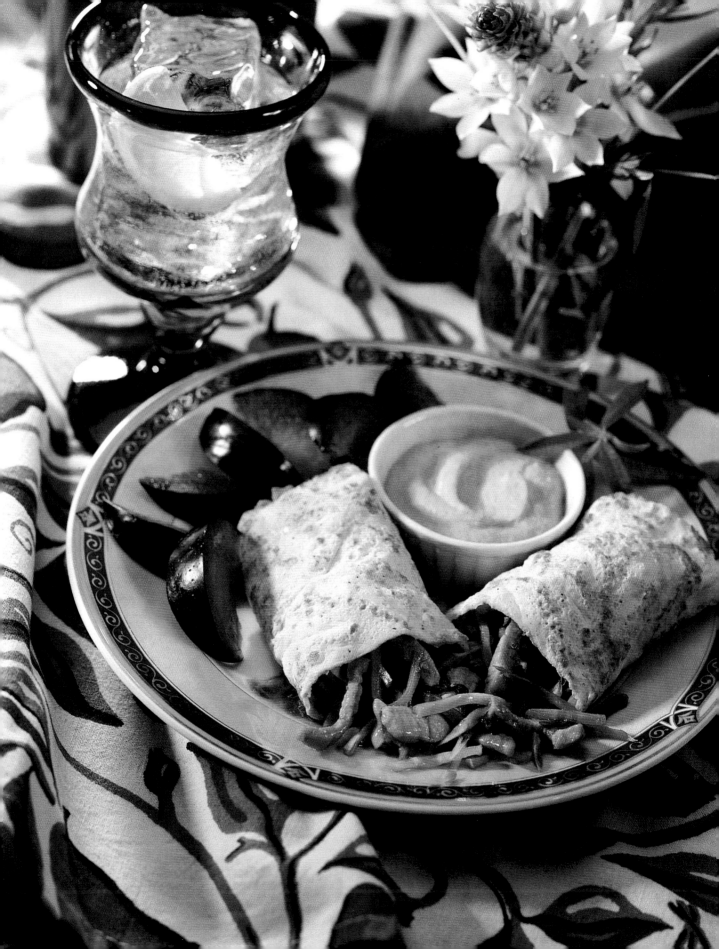

Mother Earth Pancakes

PREP: 10 min; COOK: 4 min

EIGHT 4-INCH PANCAKES

1 1/2 cups low-fat buttermilk

2 tablespoons molasses

1/4 cup fat-free cholesterol-free egg product or 2 egg whites, slightly beaten

1/2 cup all-purpose flour

1/2 cup whole wheat flour

1/4 cup wheat bran

1/2 teaspoon baking soda

Beat buttermilk, molasses and egg product in medium bowl until smooth. Stir in remaining ingredients.

Heat griddle or skillet over medium heat or to 375°; spray with nonstick cooking spray. For each pancake, pour scant 1/4 cup batter onto hot griddle. Cook pancakes until puffed and dry around edges. Turn and cook other sides until golden brown.

1 4-inch Pancake:		% Daily Value:	
Calories	90	Vitamin A	0%
Calories from fat	10	Vitamin C	0%
Fat, g	1	Calcium	6%
Saturated, g	1	Iron	6%
Cholesterol, mg	2	**Diet Exchanges:**	
Sodium, mg	140	1 starch/bread	
Carbohydrate, g	18		
Dietary Fiber, g	2		
Protein, g	4		

Stuffed French Toast

PREP: 15 min; COOK: 6 min

6 SERVINGS

Use your favorite jam or preserves in this tasty recipe.

12 slices French bread, 1/2 inch thick

6 tablespoons fat-free soft cream cheese

1/4 cup preserves or jam, any flavor

1/2 cup fat-free cholesterol-free egg product or 3 eggs whites, slightly beaten

1/2 cup skim milk

2 tablespoons granulated sugar

Powdered sugar

Maple-flavored syrup, if desired

Spread one side of each of 6 slices bread with 1 tablespoon of the cream cheese. Spread one side of each of the remaining slices with 2 teaspoons of the marmalade. Place bread with cream cheese and bread with marmalade together in pairs. Beat egg product, milk and granulated sugar until smooth; pour into shallow bowl.

Spray griddle or skillet with non-stick cooking spray; heat griddle or skillet over medium-low heat or to 325°. Dip each side of sandwich into egg mixture. Cook sandwiches 2 to 3 minutes on each side or until golden brown. Transfer to plate; dust with powdered sugar. Serve with syrup.

1 Serving:		% Daily Value:	
Calories	260	Vitamin A	4%
Calories from fat	45	Vitamin C	0%
Fat, g	5	Calcium	8%
Saturated, g	2	Iron	10%
Cholesterol, mg	5	**Diet Exchanges:**	
Sodium, mg	420	2 starch/bread	
Carbohydrate, g	47	1 fruit	
Dietary Fiber, g	2	1 fat	
Protein, g	8		

Wake-Up Shake

PREP: 5 min

2 SERVINGS (ABOUT 1 CUP EACH)

1 cup vanilla fat-free yogurt

1/2 cup frozen berries (such as raspberries or blueberries)

1/4 cup orange juice

1 medium banana, cut into chunks

Place all ingredients in blender. Cover and blend on high speed about 30 seconds or until smooth. Serve immediately.

1 Serving:		% Daily Value:	
Calories	215	Vitamin A	10%
Calories from fat	10	Vitamin C	46%
Fat, g	1	Calcium	18%
Saturated, g	1	Iron	8%
Cholesterol, mg	2	**Diet Exchanges:**	
Sodium, mg	55	3 fruit	
Carbohydrate, g	49	1/2 skim milk	
Dietary Fiber, g	4		
Protein, g	6		

Banana-Peach Shake

PREP: 5 min

3 SERVINGS (ABOUT 3/4 CUP EACH)

This breakfast is a great way to use up those overripe bananas! You can always mash bananas and freeze in ice-cube trays about 2 hours or until frozen, then transfer to freezer bags, so you'll always have them on hand for this refreshing shake. The recipe can be easily doubled for times you'd like more than three servings.

1 cup mashed ripe bananas (2 large), frozen

1 cup peach or apricot nectar

1/2 cup skim milk

Place all ingredients in blender. Cover and blend on high speed about 30 seconds or until smooth. Serve immediately over ice cubes.

1 Serving:		% Daily Value:	
Calories	125	Vitamin A	4%
Calories from fat	0	Vitamin C	18%
Fat, g	0	Calcium	6%
Saturated, g	0	Iron	2%
Cholesterol, mg	0	**Diet Exchanges:**	
Sodium, mg	30	2 fruit	
Carbohydrate, g	31		
Dietary Fiber, g	2		
Protein, g	2		

Morning Parfaits

PREP: 10 min

2 SERVINGS

Summer fresh fruits make these parfaits delicious and refreshing.

1 cup vanilla fat-free yogurt

1/8 teaspoon almond extract

1/3 cup chopped cantaloupe

1/3 cup chopped strawberries

1/3 cup chopped kiwifruit

2 tablespoons sliced almonds, toasted

Mix yogurt and almond extract. Alternate layers of fruit and 1/4 cup yogurt mixture in 2 goblets or parfait glasses, beginning and ending with fruit. Top with almonds.

1 Serving:		% Daily Value:	
Calories	160	Vitamin A	18%
Calories from fat	35	Vitamin C	96%
Fat, g	4	Calcium	18%
Saturated, g	1	Iron	8%
Cholesterol, mg	2	**Diet Exchanges:**	
Sodium, mg	55	1 1/2 fruit	
Carbohydrate, g	26	1/2 skim milk	
Dietary Fiber, g	2	1/2 fat	
Protein, g	7		

Fresh Fruit Bruschetta

PREP: 10 min

4 SERVINGS

Mix your favorite fruit with yogurt, and spoon onto a bagel—the perfect breakfast to eat on the go!

1/3 cup diced banana

1/3 cup chopped fresh or canned (drained) peaches

1/3 cup raspberries

1/4 cup vanilla, lemon or Key lime low-fat yogurt

2 soft bagels, split in half, or 4 slices banana bread, 1/2 inch thick

1 tablespoon prepared cinnamon-sugar

Mix banana, peaches, raspberries and yogurt. Toast bagels. Sprinkle cinnamon-sugar evenly over warm bagel halves. Top each bagel half with 1/4 cup fruit mixture.

1 Serving:		% Daily Value:	
Calories	125	Vitamin A	0%
Calories from fat	10	Vitamin C	8%
Fat, g	1	Calcium	4%
Saturated, g	0	Iron	6%
Cholesterol, mg	0	**Diet Exchanges:**	
Sodium, mg	160	1 starch/bread	
Carbohydrate, g	27	1 fruit	
Dietary Fiber, g	2		
Protein, g	4		

Fresh Fruit Bruschetta

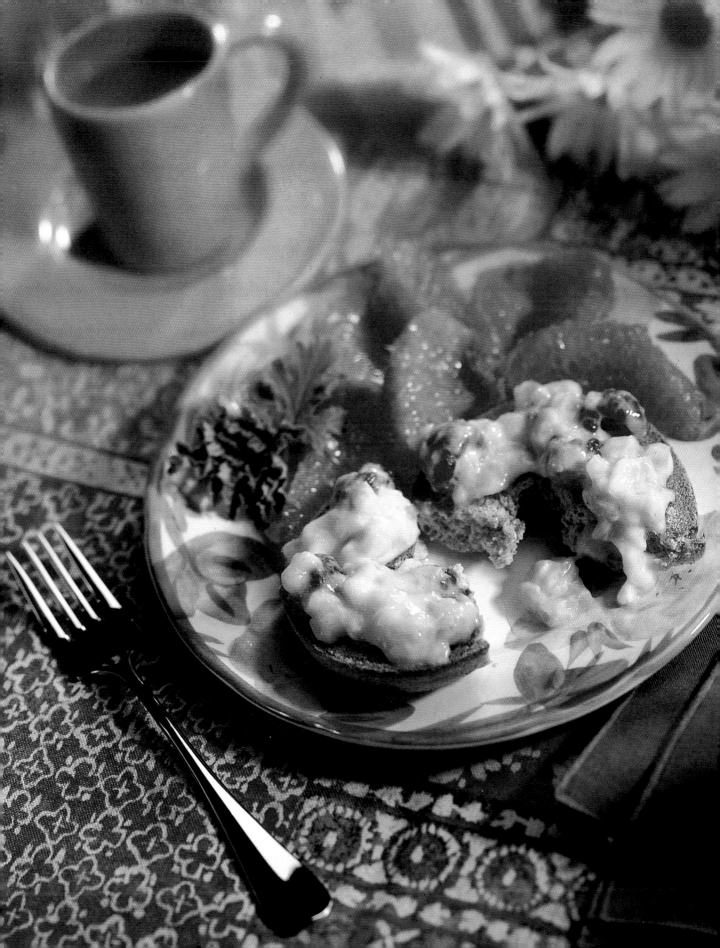

Muffin Mania

Muffins, muffins everywhere! It's not just blueberry or bran muffins anymore—now we have chocolate chocolate-chip, apricot white-chocolate chunk and strawberry cream cheese flavors to choose from in bakeries, stores and restaurants. These muffins are usually larger or jumbo in size compared to homemade muffins.

For many, a muffin seems like a healthful breakfast choice over a sweet roll, doughnut or even a scrambled egg. It may surprise you to learn how high in fat and calories muffins can be. Take a look at how those large-sized muffins measure up. You may feel inspired to change your muffin habits!

Muffin Flavor	Calories	Fat (grams)
Apple	540	24
Banana	586	29
Blueberry	506	23
Bran	478	17
Carrot	560	23
Chocolate Chocolate-Chip	546	26
Corn	683	17
Cranberry	558	28

Other Breakfast Favorites

Food	Calories	Fat (grams)
Plain cake doughnut	100	5
Plain croissant	310	19
Caramel roll	385	18
English muffin with honey	130	1
Bagel with cream cheese	250	10
Toast (2 slices) with butter and jam	178	3
Bowl of toasted oat cereal with milk	155	1.5
Egg, cheese and ham on muffin from fast-food restaurant	280	11

Mango-Lime Muffins

PREP: 10 min; BAKE: 18 min

12 MUFFINS

The skin of mangoes is thin, tough and green. As mangoes ripen, the skin becomes yellow with red mottling; to ripen a mango, place it in a paper bag at room temperature. Ripe mangoes can be placed in a plastic bag and refrigerated for up to 5 days. They add a wonderful exotic taste to these muffins.

1/4 cup fat-free cholesterol-free egg product

2 cups Bisquick® Reduced Fat baking mix

1/3 cup sugar

1 tablespoon grated lime peel

2/3 cup skim milk

2 tablespoons vegetable oil

1 cup chopped mango, peach or nectarine

Heat oven to 400°. Line 12 medium muffin cups, 2 1/2×1 1/4 inches, with paper baking cups. Beat egg product slightly in medium bowl. Stir in baking mix, sugar, lime peel, milk and oil just until moistened. Stir in mango.

Divide batter evenly among muffin cups. Bake 15 to 18 minutes or until golden brown. Immediately remove from pan to wire rack. Serve warm if desired.

1 Muffin:		% Daily Value:	
Calories	130	Vitamin A	6%
Calories from fat	35	Vitamin C	2%
Fat, g	4	Calcium	4%
Saturated, g	1	Iron	4%
Cholesterol, mg	0	**Diet Exchanges:**	
Sodium, mg	230	1 starch/bread	
Carbohydrate, g	22	1/2 fruit	
Dietary Fiber, g	0	1/2 fat	
Protein, g	2		

Lemon–Poppy Seed Scones

PREP: 10 min; BAKE: 15 min

8 SCONES

2 cups all-purpose flour

3 teaspoons baking powder

1/4 teaspoon salt

1/4 cup sugar

1 tablespoon poppy seed

1/3 cup stick margarine

2 tablespoons lemon juice

3/4 cup skim milk

Sugar, if desired

Heat oven to 425°. Spray cookie sheet with nonstick cooking spray. Mix flour, baking powder, salt, 1/4 cup sugar and the poppy seed in large bowl. Cut in margarine, using pastry blender or crisscrossing 2 knives, until mixture resembles fine crumbs. Mix lemon juice and milk; stir into flour mixture until dough leaves side of bowl and forms a ball.

Turn dough onto lightly floured surface; gently roll in flour to coat. Knead lightly 10 times. Roll or pat into 9-inch circle. Sprinkle with sugar. Cut into 8 wedges. Place on cookie sheet. Bake 12 to 15 minutes or until golden brown. Immediately remove from cookie sheet. Serve warm.

1 Scone:		% Daily Value:	
Calories	210	Vitamin A	12%
Calories from fat	70	Vitamin C	0%
Fat, g	8	Calcium	14%
Saturated, g	2	Iron	10%
Cholesterol, mg	0	**Diet Exchanges:**	
Sodium, mg	360	2 starch/bread	
Carbohydrate, g	32	1 fat	
Dietary Fiber, g	1		
Protein, g	4		

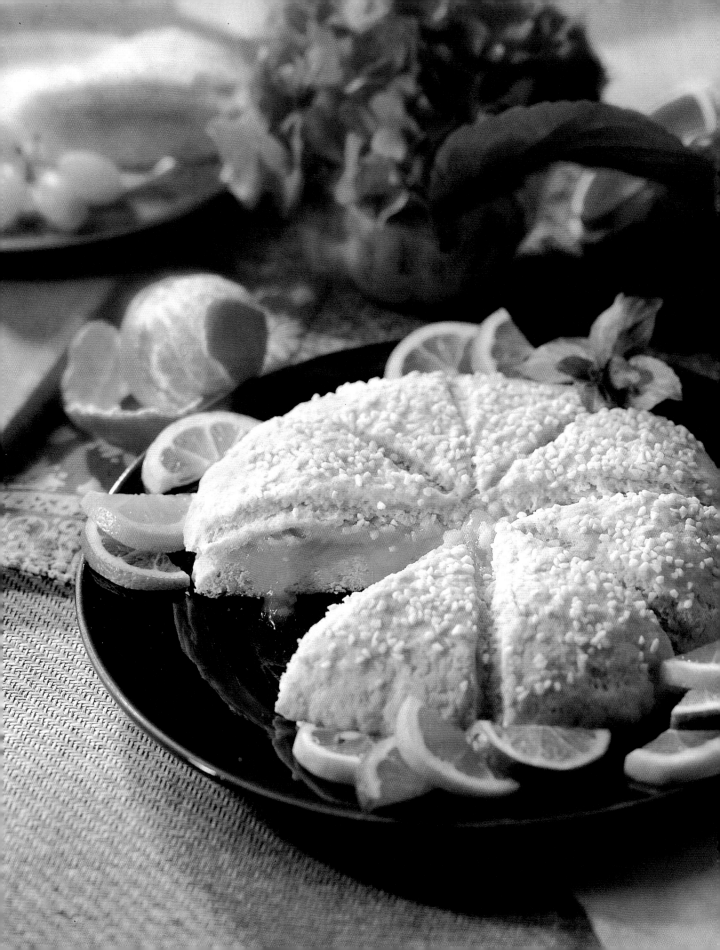

Lemon-Filled Fresh Ginger Scones

PREP: 20 min; BAKE: 20 min

8 SERVINGS

Lemon curd is often used to fill pastries, as well as a spread for bread. Prepared lemon curd is available in most large supermarkets and specialty gourmet shops.

2 cups all-purpose flour

1/4 cup sugar

3 teaspoons baking powder

1/3 cup stick margarine

2/3 cup fat-free buttermilk

1 tablespoon grated gingerroot

1/2 cup lemon curd

Sugar, if desired

Heat oven to 400°. Spray cookie sheet with non-stick cooking spray. Mix flour, sugar and baking powder in large bowl. Cut in margarine using pastry blender or crisscrossing 2 knives, until mixture resembles fine crumbs. Stir in buttermilk and gingerroot until dough leaves side of bowl and forms a ball.

Divide dough in half. Place half of dough on cookie sheet; pat or roll into 7-inch circle. Spread lemon curd over dough to within 1/2 inch of edge. Pat or roll remaining dough into 7-inch circle; gently place over lemon curd. Gently pinch edge to seal. Sprinkle with sugar. Cut surface of dough into 8 wedges, making cuts 1/4 inch deep (do not cut into lemon curd). Bake 18 to 20 minutes or until golden brown. Cool 5 minutes. Cut into wedges. Serve warm.

1 Serving:		% Daily Value:	
Calories	270	Vitamin A	10%
Calories from fat	80	Vitamin C	0%
Fat, g	9	Calcium	12%
Saturated, g	2	Iron	8%
Cholesterol, mg	0	**Diet Exchanges:**	
Sodium, mg	310	3 starch/bread	
Carbohydrate, g	44	1 fat	
Dietary Fiber, g	1		
Protein, g	4		

Lemon-Filled Fresh Ginger Scones

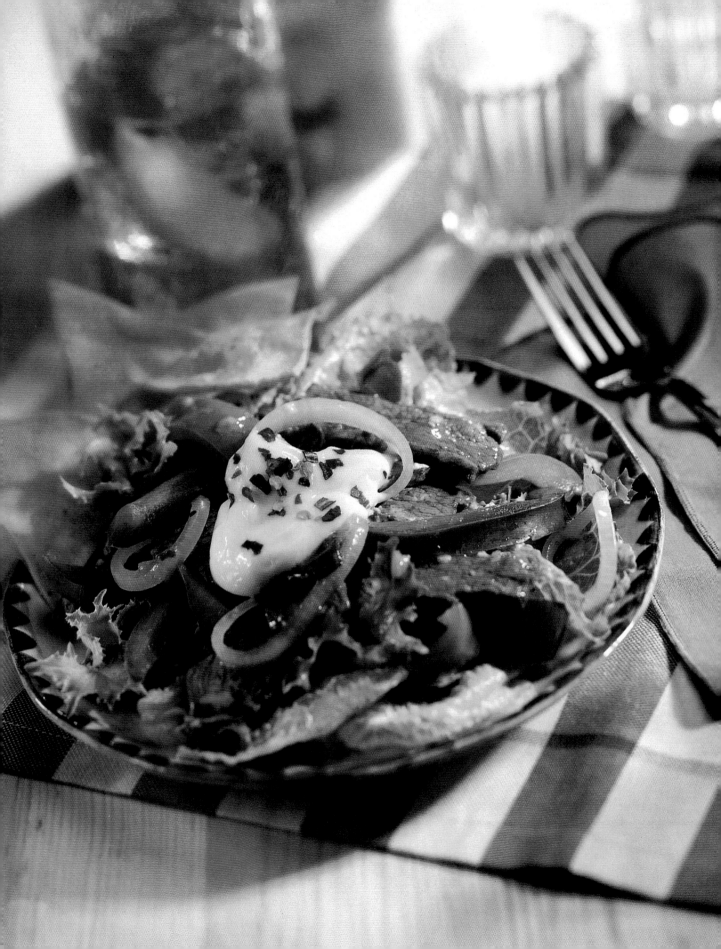

3

Hearty Soups, Salads and Sandwiches

Fajita Salad
(page 79)

Pasta and Kidney Bean Soup

PREP: 10 min; COOK: 40 min

4 SERVINGS

1/2 cup chopped red onion

1 can (14 1/2 ounces) whole tomatoes, undrained

4 cups ready-to-serve fat-free reduced-sodium chicken broth

1 cup uncooked rosamarina (orzo) pasta

1 tablespoon chopped fresh or 1/2 teaspoon dried oregano leaves

1/8 teaspoon crushed red pepper

1 clove garlic, crushed

1 can (15 to 16 ounces) red kidney beans, rinsed and drained

2 tablespoons grated fat-free Parmesan cheese

Spray 3-quart saucepan with nonstick cooking spray. Cook onion in saucepan over medium heat about 10 minutes, stirring frequently, until tender. Stir in and break up tomatoes. Stir in broth, pasta, oregano, red pepper and garlic. Heat to boiling; reduce heat to low. Cover and simmer about 20 minutes, stirring occasionally, until pasta is tender.

Stir in beans. Simmer uncovered about 10 minutes or until beans are hot. Sprinkle with cheese.

1 Serving:		% Daily Value:	
Calories	235	Vitamin A	6%
Calories from fat	20	Vitamin C	14%
Fat, g	2	Calcium	10%
Saturated, g	1	Iron	22%
Cholesterol, mg	2	**Diet Exchanges:**	
Sodium, mg	960	3 starch/bread	
Carbohydrate, g	47		
Dietary Fiber, g	6		
Protein, g	13		

Stir-Fried Beef and Vegetable Soup

PREP: 10 min; COOK: 10 min

6 SERVINGS

This quick and easy one-dish meal lets you have a healthy dinner, even on the busiest night!

1 tablespoon vegetable oil

1/2 pound beef boneless sirloin steak, thinly sliced

1 package (16 ounces) refrigerated chopped vegetables for stir-fry

1 package (about 7 ounces) fresh (refrigerated) stir-fry noodles with soy sauce-flavored sauce

1 can (14 1/2 ounces) ready-to-serve Oriental or beef broth

3 cups water

Heat oil in Dutch oven over medium-high heat. Cook beef in oil about 2 minutes, stirring occasionally, until brown. Stir in remaining ingredients; heat to boiling. Boil about 5 minutes, stirring occasionally, until vegetables are crisp-tender.

1 Serving:		% Daily Value:	
Calories	155	Vitamin A	12%
Calories from fat	35	Vitamin C	8%
Fat, g	4	Calcium	0%
Saturated, g	1	Iron	8%
Cholesterol, mg	20	**Diet Exchanges:**	
Sodium, mg	440	1 starch/bread	
Carbohydrate, g	20	1 lean meat	
Dietary Fiber, g	2	1 vegetable	
Protein, g	12		

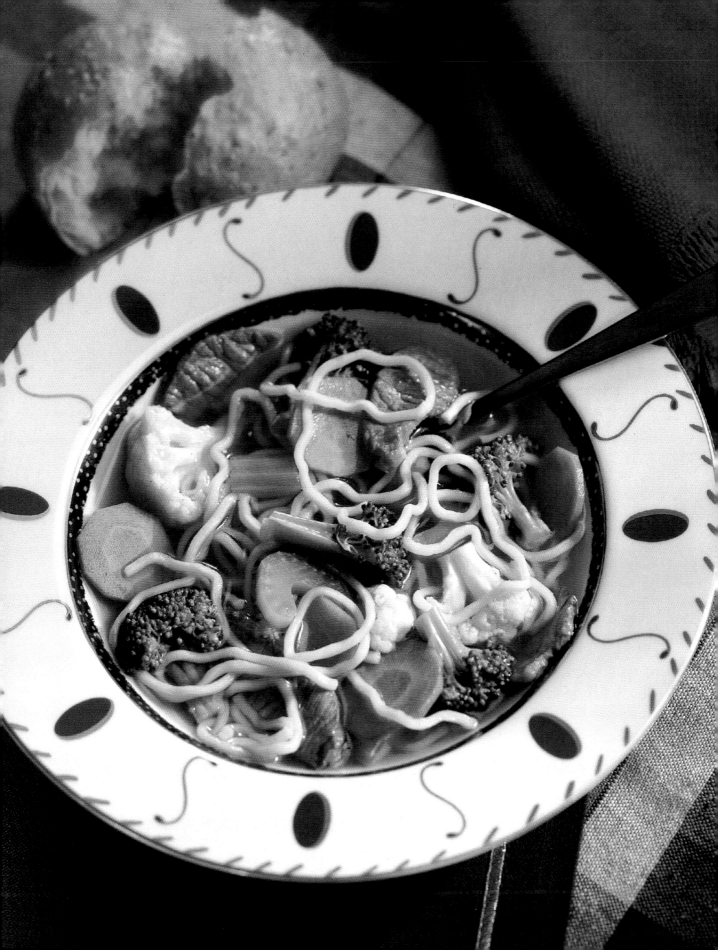

Chunky Chili Soup

PREP: 5 min; COOK: 12 min

5 SERVINGS

1/2 pound extra-lean ground beef

1 tablespoon instant minced onion

1 can (15 to 16 ounces) red kidney beans, undrained

1 can (10 3/4 ounces) condensed reduced-fat tomato soup

1 soup can water

2 to 3 teaspoons chili powder

Cook beef and onion in 2-quart saucepan over medium-high heat, stirring occasionally, until beef is brown; drain. Stir in remaining ingredients. Heat to boiling, stirring occasionally.

1 Serving:		% Daily Value:	
Calories	175	Vitamin A	4%
Calories from fat	55	Vitamin C	0%
Fat, g	6	Calcium	2%
Saturated, g	2	Iron	14%
Cholesterol, mg	25	**Diet Exchanges:**	
Sodium, mg	470	1 starch/bread	
Carbohydrate, g	20	1 medium-fat meat	
Dietary Fiber, g	4	1 fat	
Protein, g	14		

Creamy Vegetable-Cheese Soup

PREP: 5 min; COOK: 10 min

8 SERVINGS

4 ounces fat-free process cheese product loaf, cubed

3 1/2 cups skim milk

1/2 teaspoon chili powder

2 cups cooked brown or white rice

1 package (16 ounces) frozen cauliflower, carrots and asparagus, thawed and drained

Heat cheese and milk in 3-quart saucepan or Dutch oven over low heat, stirring frequently, until cheese is melted. Stir in chili powder. Stir in rice and vegetables; heat through.

1 Serving:		% Daily Value:	
Calories	125	Vitamin A	30%
Calories from fat	10	Vitamin C	16%
Fat, g	1	Calcium	20%
Saturated, g	0	Iron	2%
Cholesterol, mg	5	**Diet Exchanges:**	
Sodium, mg	270	1 starch/bread	
Carbohydrate, g	21	1/2 skim milk	
Dietary Fiber, g	2		
Protein, g	10		

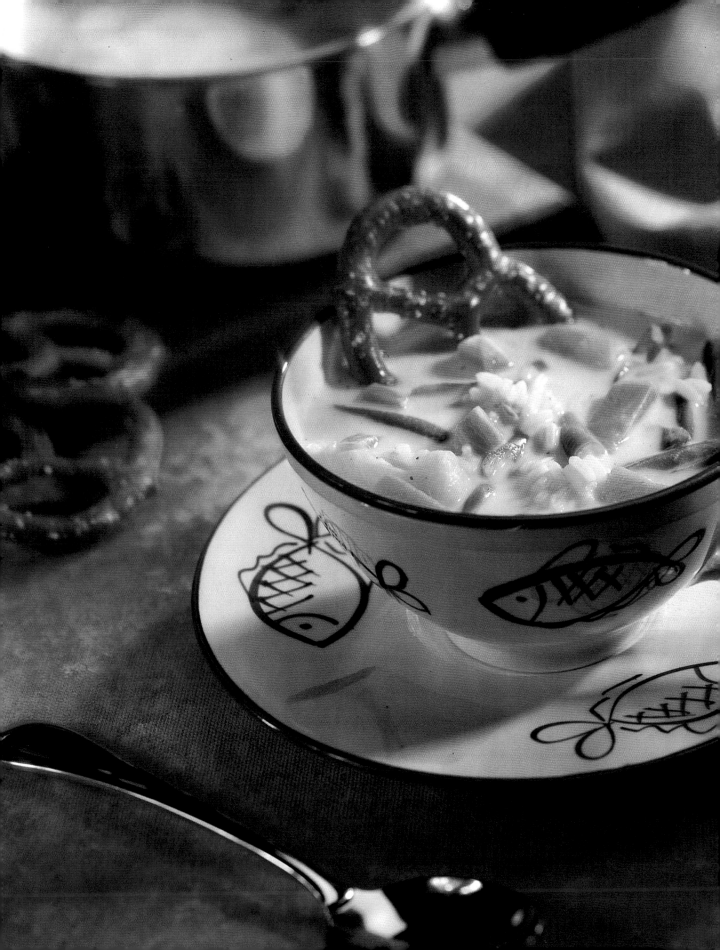

Hearty Turkey-Barley Soup

PREP: 5 min; COOK: 33 min

6 SERVINGS

Using quick-cooking barley really saves time, taking 10 to 12 minutes to cook, versus 45 to 50 minutes for regular barley.

1 pound ground turkey breast

2/3 cup uncooked quick-cooking barley

2 cans (14 1/2 ounces each) ready-to-serve beef broth

1 can (16 ounces) whole tomatoes, undrained

1 jar (23 to 24 ounces) pepper steak or cacciatore sauce

2 cups frozen mixed vegetables

Cook turkey in Dutch oven over medium heat, stirring occasionally, until no longer pink; drain. Stir in barley, broth, tomatoes and pepper steak sauce, breaking up tomatoes. Heat to boiling, stirring occasionally; reduce heat to low. Cover and simmer 15 minutes.

Stir in frozen vegetables. Cover and simmer about 10 minutes or until barley is tender.

1 Serving:		% Daily Value:	
Calories	300	Vitamin A	32%
Calories from fat	90	Vitamin C	10%
Fat, g	10	Calcium	6%
Saturated, g	3	Iron	16%
Cholesterol, mg	50	**Diet Exchanges:**	
Sodium, mg	1050	2 starch/bread	
Carbohydrate, g	36	2 lean meat	
Dietary Fiber, g	7	1 vegetable	
Protein, g	24		

Mexican Chicken-Potato Salad

PREP: 10 min; COOK: 15 min; CHILL: 1 hr

6 SERVINGS

You can use leftover, deli or canned chicken in this zesty recipe.

6 to 8 small red potatoes (1 pound), cut into fourths

1/2 cup salsa

2 cups chopped cooked chicken breast

1/2 cup fat-free mayonnaise or salad dressing

1/4 cup shredded reduced-fat Cheddar or Monterey Jack cheese (1 ounce)

6 medium green onions, sliced (3/4 cup)

1 medium jicama, peeled and cut into 1/2-inch pieces (1 cup)

1 medium stalk celery, sliced (1/2 cup)

Heat 1 inch water to boiling in 2-quart saucepan. Add potatoes. Heat to boiling; reduce heat to medium. Cover and cook 8 to 12 minutes or until tender; drain.

Reserve 2 tablespoons of the salsa. Mix potatoes, remaining salsa and remaining ingredients. Drizzle salad with reserved salsa. Cover and refrigerate at least 1 hour to blend flavors.

1 Serving:		% Daily Value:	
Calories	285	Vitamin A	2%
Calories from fat	25	Vitamin C	68%
Fat, g	3	Calcium	8%
Saturated, g	1	Iron	16%
Cholesterol, mg	35	**Diet Exchanges:**	
Sodium, mg	390	2 starch/bread	
Carbohydrate, g	38	2 lean meat	
Dietary Fiber, g	8	1 vegetable	
Protein, g	18		

Fast Food Comparisons

Either by choice or by circumstance, we often find ourselves eating at fast food restaurants. Whether for health reasons or weight loss, trying to choose the healthiest foods to order can be a guessing game. Most restaurants have complete nutrition information available upon request and employees may be able to tell you which menu item is lowest in calories and fat. This handy guide lists the most common fast foods and provides calories and fat for each. A range is given due to variances between restaurants and product weight. You may want to photocopy this list and keep a copy in the glove compartment of the car for handy reference.

Fast Food Choice	Calories	Fat(g)
Hamburgers		
Hamburger	255–340	9–15
1/4 lb. cheeseburger	390–510	23–28
1/4 lb. hamburger	344–410	19–20
Cheeseburger	305–318	13–15
"Lean" hamburger	130	7
Roast Beef Sandwiches		
Roast beef sandwich, regular size	270–383	11–18.2
Roast beef sandwich, small size	233–260	10.8–14
Light roast beef sandwich	294	10
Hot Dogs		
Hot dog	280	16
Hot dog with cheese	330	21
Hot dog with chili	320	19
Fish		
Fried fish sandwich	323–534	10–32
Baked fish fillet	151–170	1–2

(continued on next page)

Fast Food Comparisons (cont'd)

Fast Food Choice	Calories	Fat(g)
Chicken		
Fried chicken fillet sandwich	380–685	13–40
Fried chicken nuggets or tenders (6 pieces)	236–451	13–20
Grilled chicken fillet sandwich	258–451	5–19
Roast chicken sandwich	276	7
Rotisserie-style		
chicken, white meat quarter		
without skin and wing	190–242	6–9
chicken, dark meat quarter		
without skin and wing	217	10–12.2
Fried chicken pieces (with skin)		
Breast	278–412	15–27
Leg	147–190	7–11
Thigh	306–370	15–27
Fried chicken pieces (without skin)		
Breast	280–293	15–17
Leg	110–166	6–9
Thigh	256–296	17–20

Mexican

Fast Food Choice	Calories	Fat(g)
Burritos		
Bean	249–447	6–14
Beef	355–493	18–21
Chicken	227–334	10–12
Light burritos (various fillings)	330–440	6–9
Enchilada	379	18
Tacos		
Hard	183	11
Soft	225	12
Light hard	140	5
Light soft	180	5
Taco salad	450–905	18–61
Nachos	346–407	18–19

(continued on next page)

Fast Food Comparisons (cont'd)

Fast Food Choice	Calories	Fat(g)
Submarine Sandwiches		
Submarine sandwiches (6-inch size)		
Mixed cold cuts	427	20
Roast beef	375	11
Turkey	357	10
Tuna salad	402	13
Seafood salad	388	12
Vegetable	268	8.5
Pizza (1 slice from medium pizza, thin crust)		
Cheese	210–223	7–10
Sausage	282	17
Pepperoni	230	11
Sausage and pepperoni	297	16
Vegetable	192	8

SALAD BARS— THE FAT ADDS UP

All those delicious toppings are tempting. But look out! Some of your favorites are high in fat.

- 1/4 cup of Cheddar cheese has 10 grams of fat.

- 1/2 cup of creamy coleslaw has 15 grams of fat.

- 1 tablespoon of ranch dressing has 8 grams of fat.

- 1 tablespoon of sunflower seeds has 16 grams of fat.

- 6 flavored croutons have 1.5 grams of fat and 35 calories.

- 2 tablespoons of bacon bits have 3 grams of fat.

- 1/4 cup of chopped egg has 5 grams of fat.

- 2 tablespoons of raisins have 65 calories.

- 1/2 cup garbanzo beans has 142 calories.

- 1/2 cup potato salad has 179 calories.

Raspberry-Chicken Salad

PREP: 10 min

4 SERVINGS

6 cups bite-size pieces mixed salad greens (such as Bibb, iceberg, Romaine or spinach)

2 cups cut-up cooked chicken breast

1 cup raspberries*

1/3 cup thinly sliced celery

Raspberry Dressing (below)

Freshly ground pepper

Toss salad greens, chicken, raspberries and celery. Serve with Raspberry Dressing and pepper.

RASPBERRY DRESSING

1 cup plain fat-free yogurt

1/2 cup raspberries*

1 tablespoon raspberry or red wine vinegar

2 teaspoons sugar

Place all ingredients in blender. Cover and blend on high speed about 15 seconds or until smooth.

Frozen loose-pack unsweetened raspberries can be substituted for the fresh raspberries.

1 Serving:		% Daily Value:	
Calories	165	Vitamin A	2%
Calories from fat	25	Vitamin C	24%
Fat, g	3	Calcium	16%
Saturated, g	1	Iron	8%
Cholesterol, mg	55	**Diet Exchanges:**	
Sodium, mg	110	2 lean meat	
Carbohydrate, g	14	1 fruit	
Dietary Fiber, g	4		
Protein, g	25		

Raspberry-Chicken Salad

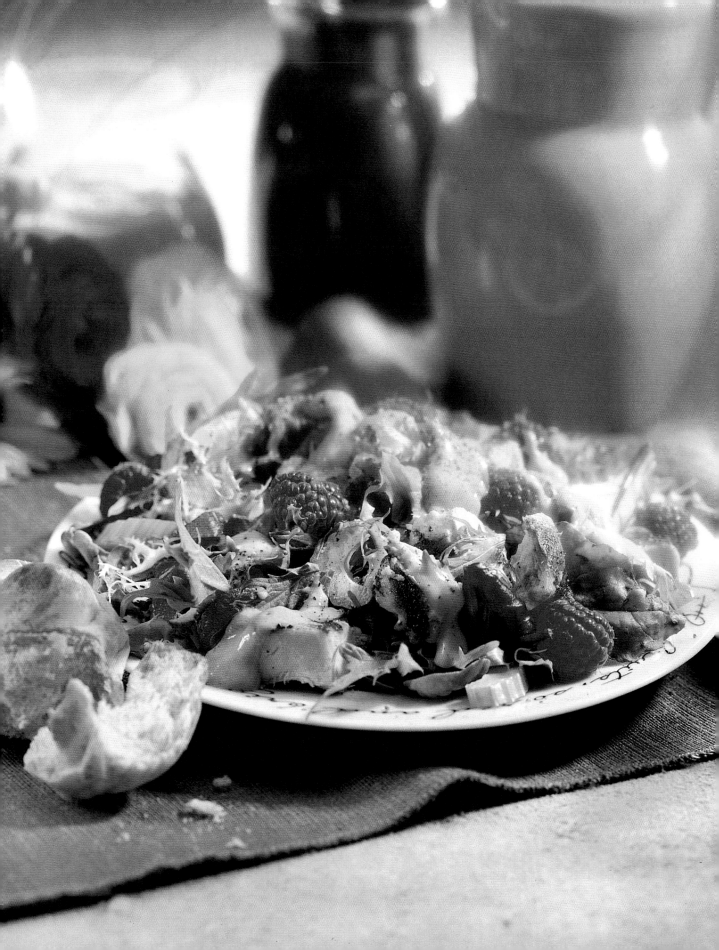

Turkey-Macaroni Salad

PREP: 12 min; CHILL 2 hr

6 SERVINGS

1 1/2 cups uncooked elbow macaroni (6 ounces)

1 package (10 ounces) frozen green peas

2 cups cut-up cooked turkey breast

3/4 cup reduced-fat mayonnaise or salad dressing

1/2 cup shredded reduced-fat Cheddar cheese (2 ounces)

1/4 cup sweet pickle relish

4 medium green onions, sliced (1/2 cup)

1 medium stalk celery, sliced (1/2 cup)

3 cups bite-size pieces lettuce (1/2 medium head)

Cook and drain macaroni as directed on package. Rinse with cold water; drain. Rinse frozen peas with cold water to separate; drain.

Mix macaroni, peas and remaining ingredients except lettuce. Cover and refrigerate 2 to 4 hours to blend flavors. Serve on lettuce.

1 Serving:		% Daily Value:	
Calories	265	Vitamin A	6%
Calories from fat	35	Vitamin C	6%
Fat, g	4	Calcium	10%
Saturated, g	2	Iron	14%
Cholesterol, mg	40	**Diet Exchanges:**	
Sodium, mg	590	2 starch/bread	
Carbohydrate, g	39	1 lean meat	
Dietary Fiber, g	4	2 vegetable	
Protein, g	22		

Beef-Macaroni Salad

PREP: 15 min

4 SERVINGS

1 package (7 ounces) elbow macaroni (2 cups)

1 cup cherry tomato halves

1 cup broccoli flowerets

3/4 cup cut-up cooked lean beef

1/2 cup coarsely chopped unpeeled cucumber

1 medium carrot, thinly sliced (1/2 cup)

1 bottle (8 ounces) fat-free creamy Italian dressing

Salad greens, if desired

Cook and drain macaroni as directed on package. Rinse with cold water; drain. Mix macaroni and remaining ingredients except salad greens. Serve on salad greens.

1 Serving:		% Daily Value:	
Calories	270	Vitamin A	34%
Calories from fat	20	Vitamin C	46%
Fat, g	2	Calcium	2%
Saturated, g	1	Iron	18%
Cholesterol, mg	20	**Diet Exchanges:**	
Sodium, mg	480	3 starch/bread	
Carbohydrate, g	50	1 vegetable	
Dietary Fiber, g	3		
Protein, g	16		

Fajita Salad

PREP: 12 min; COOK: 6 min

4 SERVINGS

3/4 pound lean beef boneless sirloin steak

2 teaspoons vegetable oil

2 medium bell peppers, cut into strips

1 small onion, thinly sliced

4 cups bite-size pieces salad greens

1/3 cup fat-free Italian dressing

1/4 cup plain fat-free yogurt

Baked tortilla chips, if desired

Trim fat from beef if necessary. Cut beef with grain into 2-inch strips; cut strips across grain into 1/8-inch slices.

Heat oil in 10-inch nonstick skillet over medium-high heat. Cook beef in oil about 3 minutes, stirring occasionally, until no longer pink. Remove beef from skillet. Add bell peppers and onion to skillet. Cook about 3 minutes, stirring occasionally, until bell peppers are crisp-tender. Stir in beef.

Place salad greens on serving platter. Top with beef mixture. Pour dressing over salad. Top with yogurt. Serve with tortilla chips.

1 Serving:		% Daily Value:	
Calories	150	Vitamin A	4%
Calories from fat	45	Vitamin C	30%
Fat, g	5	Calcium	4%
Saturated, g	3	Iron	12%
Cholesterol, mg	45	**Diet Exchanges:**	
Sodium, mg	200	2 lean meat	
Carbohydrate, g	8	2 vegetable	
Dietary Fiber, g	1		
Protein, g	19		

California Club Pasta Salad

PREP: 15 min

6 SERVINGS

3 cups uncooked medium pasta shells (8 ounces)

3/4 cup fat-free ranch dressing

1 medium tomato, chopped (3/4 cup)

1/4 pound deli-style sliced fat-free ham, cut into 1/2-inch strips

1/4 pound deli-style sliced fat-free turkey, cut into 1/2-inch strips

2 medium green onions, sliced (1/4 cup)

6 cups spinach leaves

1/4 cup imitation bacon-flavored bits

Cook and drain pasta as directed on package. Rinse with cold water; drain. Toss pasta, dressing, tomato, ham, turkey and onions.

Place spinach on serving platter. Top with pasta mixture. Sprinkle with bacon bits.

1 Serving:		% Daily Value:	
Calories	240	Vitamin A	50%
Calories from fat	35	Vitamin C	42%
Fat, g	4	Calcium	10%
Saturated, g	2	Iron	22%
Cholesterol, mg	20	**Diet Exchanges:**	
Sodium, mg	890	2 starch/bread	
Carbohydrate, g	37	1 lean meat	
Dietary Fiber, g	3	1 vegetable	
Protein, g	17		

Oriental Pork Salad

PREP: 10 min; COOK: 5 min

4 SERVINGS

2 tablespoons reduced-sodium soy sauce

1 tablespoon chili puree with garlic

1 teaspoon sesame or vegetable oil

1/2 pound pork tenderloin, cut into 1 1/2×1/2-inch strips

3 cups coleslaw mix

1 small red bell pepper, cut into 1/2-inch strips

1 can (15 ounces) black beans, rinsed and drained

Mix soy sauce, chili puree and oil. Mix pork and 1 tablespoon of the soy sauce mixture; reserve remaining soy sauce mixture.

Spray 10-inch nonstick skillet with nonstick cooking spray; heat over medium-high heat. Cook pork in skillet, stirring occasionally, until no longer pink. Place pork in medium bowl. Add remaining soy sauce mixture and remaining ingredients; toss.

1 Serving:		% Daily Value:	
Calories	210	Vitamin A	8%
Calories from fat	35	Vitamin C	32%
Fat, g	4	Calcium	10%
Saturated, g	2	Iron	20%
Cholesterol, mg	35	**Diet Exchanges:**	
Sodium, mg	600	2 starch/bread	
Carbohydrate, g	30	1 lean meat	
Dietary Fiber, g	8		
Protein, g	22		

Couscous-Shrimp Salad

PREP: 10 min; COOK: 5 min; CHILL: 1 hr

4 SERVINGS

Quick-cooking types of couscous take only five minutes to prepare, and adds satisfying heft to this refreshing seafood salad.

1 cup uncooked couscous

3/4 pound cooked peeled deveined medium shrimp, thawed if frozen

2 medium tomatoes, chopped (1 1/2 cups)

4 medium green onions, sliced (1/2 cup)

1/3 cup fat-free Italian dressing

1/4 teaspoon pepper

Lettuce leaves

Cook couscous as directed on package but without salt and fat. Toss couscous and remaining ingredients except lettuce. Cover and refrigerate at least 1 hour to blend flavors. Serve on lettuce.

1 Serving:		% Daily Value:	
Calories	260	Vitamin A	10%
Calories from fat	10	Vitamin C	28%
Fat, g	1	Calcium	6%
Saturated, g	0	Iron	20%
Cholesterol, mg	165	**Diet Exchanges:**	
Sodium, mg	360	2 1/2 starch/bread	
Carbohydrate, g	42	1 lean meat	
Dietary Fiber, g	3	1 vegetable	
Protein, g	24		

BEST SALAD BAR CHOICES

Salad bars offer so much variety and are a fast way to create a meal. Although many food choices are available, some choices are better than others. With all of the tempting options, what should you choose if you want to lose?

- Pile on the plain veggies! Choose greens, cucumbers, tomatoes, carrots, celery, broccoli, cauliflower, mushrooms, sprouts, peppers, squash, water chestnuts, radishes and onions.

- Add a little protein. Choose chicken, turkey, ham, imitation crab, flaked tuna, kidney or garbanzo beans, and cottage cheese.

- Choose fresh fruit such as pineapple, melon, bananas and apples.

- Avoid marinated or mayonnaise-based salads (unless they are made with low-fat or fat-free salad dressing or mayonnaise), cheeses, chopped egg and olives.

- Limit higher fat toppings such as croutons, shoestring potatoes, chow mein noodles, tortilla chips, sunflower seeds and bacon bits.

- Choose low-fat or fat-free salad dressing or vinegar or lemon juice. If healthful options are not available, limit dressing to 1 or 2 tablespoons.

Chutney-Chicken Pitas

PREP: 12 min

4 SANDWICHES

1 cup finely shredded cabbage

1/4 cup plain fat-free yogurt or fat-free sour cream

1/2 teaspoon sugar

1/4 teaspoon ground mustard (dry)

1/2 cup mango chutney

6 ounces deli-style sliced fat-free chicken, diced (1 cup)

2 pita breads (6 inches in diameter), cut in half to form pockets

Mix cabbage, yogurt, sugar and mustard; set aside. Heat chutney and chicken over medium heat, stirring occasionally, until hot. Fill each pita bread half with chicken mixture. Spread cabbage mixture over chicken mixture.

1 Sandwich:		% Daily Value:	
Calories	225	Vitamin A	0%
Calories from fat	65	Vitamin C	14%
Fat, g	7	Calcium	8%
Saturated, g	2	Iron	10%
Cholesterol, mg	40	**Diet Exchanges:**	
Sodium, mg	680	2 starch/bread	
Carbohydrate, g	31	1 lean meat	
Dietary Fiber, g	1		
Protein, g	10		

Turkey Pita Stack

PREP: 15 min

4 OPEN-FACE SANDWICHES

1/2 cup Almost Guacamole (page 32)

4 pita breads (6 inches in diameter)

2 cups shredded lettuce

1 medium tomato, chopped (3/4 cup)

6 ounces thinly sliced cooked turkey breast

3/4 cup shredded reduced-fat Monterey Jack cheese (3 ounces)

Creamy Salsa (below)

Spread Almost Guacamole over pita breads. Top with lettuce, tomato and turkey. Sprinkle with cheese. Top with Creamy Salsa.

CREAMY SALSA

3 tablespoons fat-free sour cream

1 tablespoon salsa

1 medium green onion, chopped (1 tablespoon)

Mix all ingredients.

1 Sandwich:		% Daily Value:	
Calories	285	Vitamin A	8%
Calories from fat	55	Vitamin C	20%
Fat, g	6	Calcium	24%
Saturated, g	3	Iron	12%
Cholesterol, mg	30	**Diet Exchanges:**	
Sodium, mg	960	2 starch/bread	
Carbohydrate, g	40	1 1/2 lean meat	
Dietary Fiber, g	2	2 vegetable	
Protein, g	20		

Spinach Turkey Calzones

PREP: 15 min; BAKE: 25 min

4 SERVINGS

A welcome low-fat version of the popular Italian sandwich!

1/2 pound ground turkey breast

1 small onion, chopped (1/4 cup)

1 cup fat-free spaghetti sauce

1 package (10 ounces) frozen chopped spinach, thawed and squeezed to drain

1/4 teaspoon pepper

1 can (10 ounces) refrigerated pizza crust dough

1/2 cup fat-free spaghetti sauce, heated

1/4 cup shredded reduced-fat mozzarella cheese (1 ounce)

Heat oven to 400°. Spray 10-inch nonstick skillet with nonstick cooking spray; heat over medium-high heat. Cook turkey and onion 5 to 6 minutes, stirring occasionally, until turkey is no longer pink; drain. Stir in 1 cup spaghetti sauce, the spinach and pepper.

Pat or roll pizza crust dough into 12-inch square. Cut into four 6-inch squares. Spoon spinach mixture onto half of each square to within 1/2 inch of edge. Fold dough over filling; press edges to seal. Place on ungreased cookie sheet. Bake about 25 minutes or until golden brown. Top each with 2 tablespoons of the heated spaghetti sauce. Sprinkle with cheese.

1 Serving:		% Daily Value:	
Calories	330	Vitamin A	50%
Calories from fat	65	Vitamin C	6%
Fat, g	7	Calcium	12%
Saturated, g	2	Iron	24%
Cholesterol, mg	35	**Diet Exchanges:**	
Sodium, mg	740	3 starch/bread	
Carbohydrate, g	49	1 lean meat	
Dietary Fiber, g	5	1 vegetable	
Protein, g	23		

Smoked Turkey and Cranberry Sandwiches

PREP: 10 min

MAKES **4** SERVINGS

Now, fat-free packages of sliced meats are available in the cold cuts section of the grocery store. Fat-free meat helps make this sandwich delicious, yet healthy.

1/3 cup fat-free cream cheese, softened

1/3 cup cranberry-orange relish or whole berry cranberry sauce

8 slices whole-grain bread

6 ounces deli-style sliced fat-free smoked turkey

4 lettuce leaves

Mix cream cheese and relish. Spread over bread slices. Place turkey and lettuce on 4 bread slices. Top with remaining bread.

1 Serving:		% Daily Value:	
Calories	225	Vitamin A	2%
Calories from fat	25	Vitamin C	8%
Fat, g	3	Calcium	8%
Saturated, g	1	Iron	10%
Cholesterol, mg	20	**Diet Exchanges:**	
Sodium, mg	910	2 starch/bread	
Carbohydrate, g	37	1 lean meat	
Dietary Fiber, g	3	1/2 fruit	
Protein, g	15		

Smoked Turkey and Cranberry Sandwiches

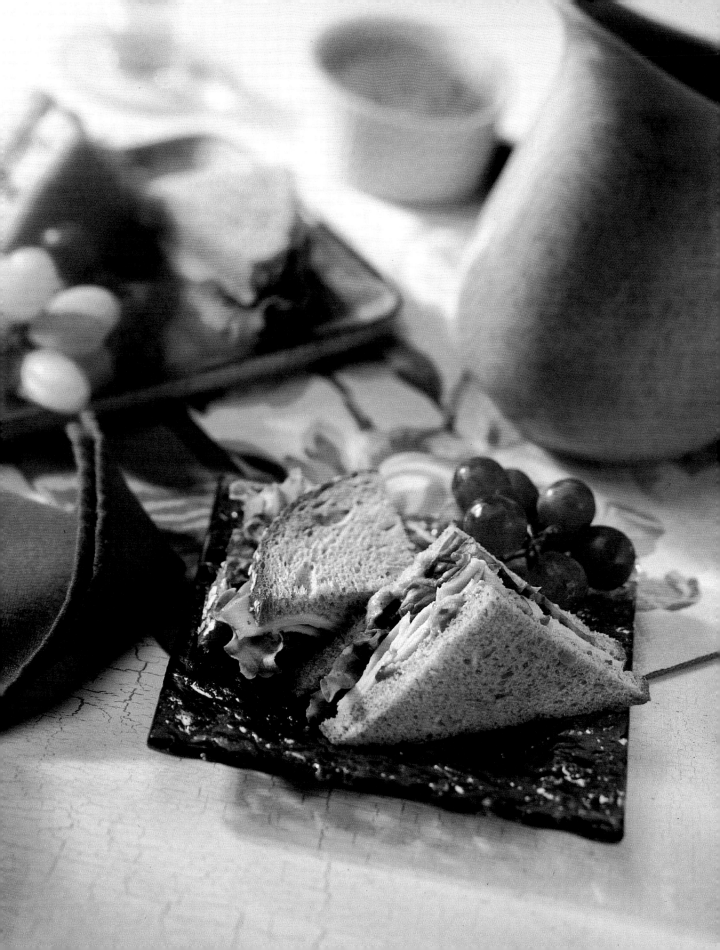

Turkey Sloppy Joes

PREP: 5 min; COOK: 12 min

6 SANDWICHES

1 pound ground turkey breast or extra-lean ground beef

1 medium onion, chopped (1/2 cup)

2 teaspoons Worcestershire sauce

3 drops red pepper sauce

1 can (10 3/4 ounces) reduced-fat condensed tomato soup

6 hamburger buns, split

Cook turkey and onion in 2-quart saucepan over medium-high heat, stirring occasionally, until turkey is no longer pink; drain.

Stir in remaining ingredients except buns. Cook, stirring occasionally, until hot. Fill buns with turkey mixture.

1 Sandwich:		% Daily Value:	
Calories	240	Vitamin A	0%
Calories from fat	45	Vitamin C	0%
Fat, g	5	Calcium	8%
Saturated, g	2	Iron	12%
Cholesterol, mg	45	**Diet Exchanges:**	
Sodium, mg	450	2 starch/bread	
Carbohydrate, g	29	1 1/2 lean meat	
Dietary Fiber, g	2		
Protein, g	22		

Roast Beef Pocket Sandwiches

PREP: 10 min

4 SANDWICHES

1 cup plain fat-free yogurt

1 1/2 teaspoons chopped fresh or 1/2 teaspoon dried dill weed

1 teaspoon mustard

1 medium bell pepper, chopped (1 cup)

2 pita breads (6 inches in diameter), cut in half to form pockets

1/3 pound thinly sliced lean roast beef

1 cup alfalfa sprouts

Mix yogurt, dill weed and mustard in small bowl. Stir in bell pepper. Fill each pita bread half with 1/3 cup yogurt mixture and one-fourth of the beef and alfalfa sprouts.

1 Sandwich:		% Daily Value:	
Calories	180	Vitamin A	0%
Calories from fat	20	Vitamin C	30%
Fat, g	2	Calcium	16%
Saturated, g	1	Iron	12%
Cholesterol, mg	35	**Diet Exchanges:**	
Sodium, mg	250	1 1/2 starch/bread	
Carbohydrate, g	23	1 lean meat	
Dietary Fiber, g	1		
Protein, g	18		

Fact Versus Fiction: Fitness Claims

Q: If I don't feel discomfort or pain, is there any benefit?

A: Exercise should not hurt. If you're feeling uncomfortable, you may be pushing yourself too hard. Choose something you enjoy and ease into it.

Q: Is it true that the more you sweat, the more fat you lose?

A: If you exercise in the heat or in a rubberized suit, you will sweat profusely and lose weight. The weight loss will be a result of lost water, not lost fat. Those pounds will return just as quickly once you replenish your body by drinking and eating. Keep in mind that how much you sweat is not a good indicator of energy expenditure. Perspiring is more dependent on factors such as temperature, humidity, body composition, lack of conditioning and individual variance.

Q: Can you burn fat from specific areas of the body by exercising those areas?

A: Contrary to popular belief, there is no such thing as "spot reduction." When exercising, your body produces energy by metabolizing fat from all regions of the body, not just from the body parts involved. For example, doing sit-ups will not trim fat from your abdomen. It will tone the muscles, but aerobic exercise is needed to burn the fat.

Q: If I don't have time for an extensive, time-consuming workout, why bother?

A: A little bit of something is better than nothing, so all those leg jigglers, toe tappers and finger rappers are burning a few more calories than someone not moving at all! Studies have shown that measurable conditioning and calorie expenditure can take place with workouts as short as fifteen minutes a couple of times a day. You don't necessarily have to change clothes and be drenched with sweat to do your body some good. Put aside a little time to start with and expand your workout as you find time or want to make more of a commitment.

Q: Is it true that weight training turns fat into muscle, so if I don't lose weight before starting a weight training program, my extra weight will turn into muscle and I won't lose the weight?

A: Fat and muscle tissue are distinctly different. One *may not* become the other. Through weight training, you will be increasing your muscle tissue, *not* turning fat into muscle. Weight training will strengthen and tone your muscles. The way to lose fat is through aerobic exercise.

Vegetable Tortillas

PREP: 10 min; COOK: 6 min

6 SERVINGS

1/2 cup diced red bell pepper

1/2 cup diced yellow bell pepper

1/2 cup diced chayote or zucchini

6 fat-free flour tortillas (6 to 8 inches in diameter)

1 1/2 cups shredded reduced-fat Monterey Jack cheese (6 ounces)

Mix bell peppers and chayote. Spoon 1/4 cup of the vegetable mixture onto center of each tortilla. Top each with 1/4 cup of the cheese. Roll tortilla tightly around vegetable mixture.

Spray 10-inch skillet with nonstick cooking spray; heat over medium heat. Cook 2 filled tortillas, seam sides down, in skillet about 3 minutes or until bottoms are light brown. Spray tops of tortillas lightly with cooking spray; turn tortillas. Cook about 3 minutes longer or until bottoms are light brown. Repeat with remaining tortillas.

1 Serving:		% Daily Value:	
Calories	190	Vitamin A	8%
Calories from fat	45	Vitamin C	26%
Fat, g	5	Calcium	20%
Saturated, g	3	Iron	0%
Cholesterol, mg	15	**Diet Exchanges:**	
Sodium, mg	490	1 starch/bread	
Carbohydrate, g	26	1 vegetable	
Dietary Fiber, g	1	1/2 skim milk	
Protein, g	11	1 fat	

Vegetable and Pork Pita Sandwiches

PREP: 15 min; BROIL: 8 min

4 SANDWICHES (2 HALVES EACH)

3 medium zucchini (1 1/2 pounds), cut into 3×1/2-inch strips

2 medium red bell peppers, cut into 1/4-inch strips

2 pork boneless loin chops (about 1/2 pound), cut into 1/4-inch strips

1/4 cup fat-free Italian dressing

1/2 teaspoon pepper

2 tablespoons grated fat-free Parmesan cheese

2 tablespoons chopped fresh parsley or 2 teaspoons dried parsley flakes

Lettuce leaves, if desired

4 whole wheat pita breads (6 inches in diameter), cut in half to form pockets

Set oven control to broil. Spray jelly roll pan, 15 1/2×10 1/2×1 inch, with nonstick cooking spray. Place zucchini, bell peppers and pork in heavy-duty resealable plastic bag. Add dressing and pepper. Seal bag; shake bag to coat ingredients. Pour mixture into pan; spread evenly.

Broil with tops 2 to 3 inches from heat 6 to 8 minutes, stirring once, until pork is no longer pink. Sprinkle with cheese and parsley. Line pita bread halves with lettuce. Spoon pork mixture into pita bread halves.

1 Sandwich:		% Daily Value:	
Calories	245	Vitamin A	28%
Calories from fat	55	Vitamin C	100%
Fat, g	6	Calcium	8%
Saturated, g	3	Iron	16%
Cholesterol, mg	35	**Diet Exchanges:**	
Sodium, mg	510	2 1/2 starch/bread	
Carbohydrate, g	42	1 lean meat	
Dietary Fiber, g	7	1 vegetable	
Protein, g	20		

Vegetable and Pork Pita Sandwiches

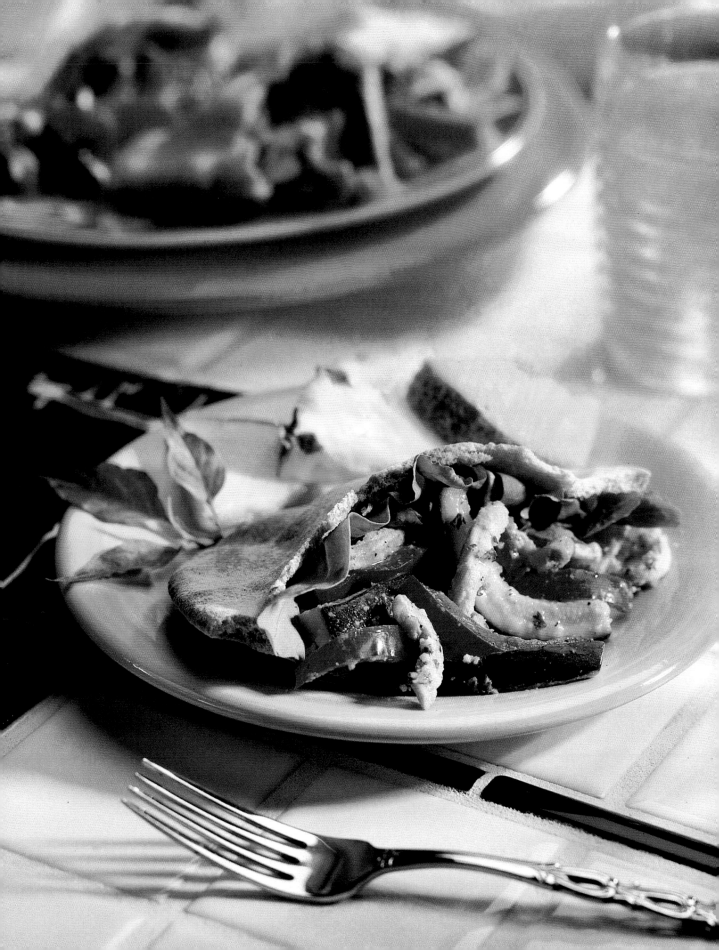

Deli Dilemma

Stopping at the deli is often a quick mealtime solution, but the large array of appetizing foods can certainly test your willpower! Knowing what foods to choose from all of those temptations will steer you in the right direction. Many delis now offer "light" selections that are lower in fat and calories, and some may offer sugar-free gelatin salads, puddings and desserts. Ask for nutrition information on the light selections so you know what you are eating.

Best Choices	Worst Choices
Light salads or entrées (check nutrition information if provided or ask about calories and fat). As a general rule of thumb, choose items under 10 grams of fat per serving.	Mayonnaise-based salads
Marinated salads are okay if you drain off all of the marinade.	Dips and spreads
Low-fat cheeses are often available and can be purchased in very small amounts, even just 1 slice.	Liver pâté
Low-fat or fat-free deli meats	Fried chicken and buffalo wings
Low-fat or fat-free dips and spreads	Egg rolls
Rotisserie chicken (do not eat skin)	Lasagna
Fresh vegetables and fruit	Macaroni and cheese
Thin crust ready-to-use pizza crusts	Strawberry or chocolate mousse
Fruit salad	Cakes, tortes and cheesecake

Simple Shrimp Fajitas

PREP: 15 min; BAKE: 15 min; COOK: 5 min

6 SERVINGS

Serve these fajitas with Almost Guacamole on page 32 and fat-free sour cream for the complete fajita experience.

6 fat-free flour tortillas (6 to 8 inches in diameter)

3/4 pound cooked peeled deveined medium shrimp, thawed if frozen, or 1 package (12 ounces) frozen cooked shrimp, thawed

1 tablespoon lime juice

1 1/2 teaspoons chopped fresh or 1/2 teaspoon dried oregano leaves

1/4 teaspoon ground cumin

1 clove garlic, finely chopped

1 cup salsa

Additional salsa, if desired

Heat oven to 250°. Wrap tortillas in aluminum foil, or place on heatproof serving plate and cover with aluminum foil. Heat in oven about 15 minutes or until warm.

Spray 10-inch skillet with nonstick cooking spray; heat over medium heat. Cook shrimp, lime juice, oregano, cumin and garlic in skillet about 5 minutes, stirring constantly, until hot.

Divide shrimp mixture evenly among tortillas. Top with 1 cup salsa. Fold one end of each tortilla up about 1 inch over filling; fold right and left sides over folded end, overlapping. Fold down remaining end. Serve with additional salsa.

1 Serving:		% Daily Value:	
Calories	170	Vitamin A	6%
Calories from fat	10	Vitamin C	8%
Fat, g	1	Calcium	4%
Saturated, g	0	Iron	12%
Cholesterol, mg	110	**Diet Exchanges:**	
Sodium, mg	580	1 1/2 starch/bread	
Carbohydrate, g	27	1 lean meat	
Dietary Fiber, g	2		
Protein, g	15		

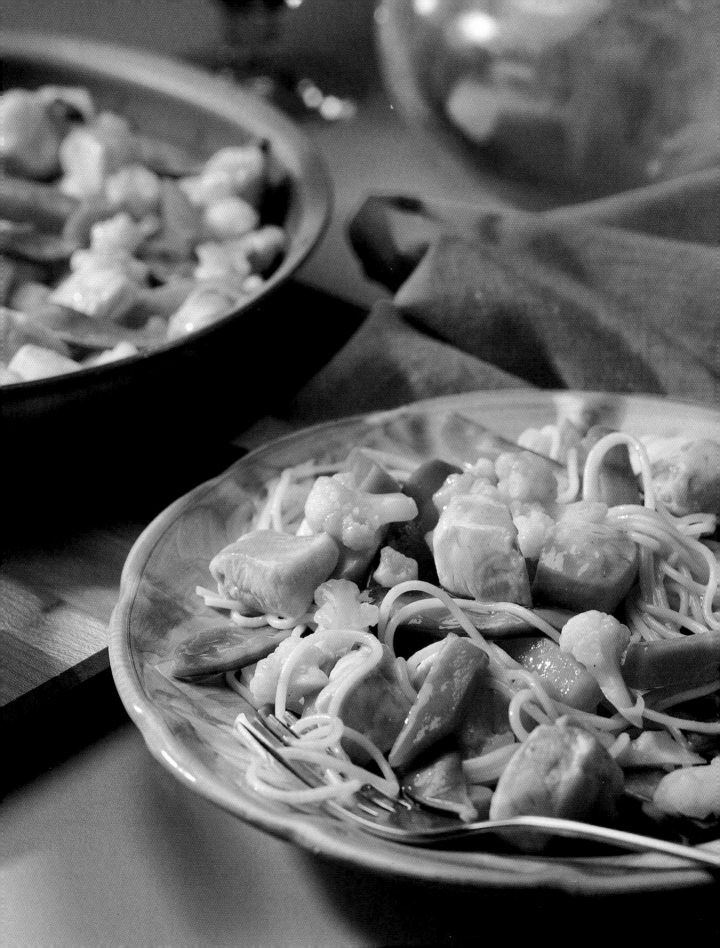

4

Easy Chicken and Turkey

Super-Easy Chicken Stir-Fry
(page 99)

Orange- and Ginger-Glazed Chicken

PREP: 5 min; COOK: 20 min

4 SERVINGS

Spreadable fruits contain no added refined sugar, but instead rely on the sugar within various fruits for sweetness.

4 skinless boneless chicken breast halves (1 pound)

1/3 cup orange marmalade spreadable fruit

1 teaspoon finely chopped gingerroot or 1/2 teaspoon ground ginger

1 teaspoon Worcestershire sauce

Spray 10-inch skillet with nonstick cooking spray; heat over medium-high heat. Cook chicken in skillet about 5 minutes or until bottoms are brown; turn chicken. Stir in remaining ingredients; reduce heat to low.

Cover and simmer 10 to 15 minutes, stirring sauce occasionally, until sauce is thickened and juice of chicken is no longer pink when centers of thickest pieces are cut. Cut chicken into thin slices. Spoon sauce over chicken.

1 Serving:		% Daily Value:	
Calories	185	Vitamin A	0%
Calories from fat	25	Vitamin C	2%
Fat, g	3	Calcium	2%
Saturated, g	1	Iron	6%
Cholesterol, mg	60	**Diet Exchanges:**	
Sodium, mg	70	2 lean meat	
Carbohydrate, g	16	1 fruit	
Dietary Fiber, g	1		
Protein, g	25		

Garlic Chicken Kiev

PREP: 30 min; FREEZE: 30 min; BAKE: 35 min

6 SERVINGS

3 tablespoons reduced-calorie spread, softened

1 tablespoon chopped fresh chives or parsley

1/8 teaspoon garlic powder

6 skinless boneless chicken breast halves (1 1/2 pounds)

2 cups cornflakes, crushed (about 1 cup)

2 tablespoons chopped fresh parsley

1/2 teaspoon paprika

1/4 cup low-fat buttermilk or skim milk

Mix spread, chives and garlic powder; shape into rectangle, 3 × 2 inches. Cover and freeze about 30 minutes or until firm.

Trim fat from chicken. Flatten each chicken breast half to 1/4-inch thickness between waxed paper or plastic wrap.

Heat oven to 425°. Spray square pan, 9 × 9 × 2 inches, with nonstick cooking spray. Cut chives mixture crosswise into 6 pieces. Place 1 piece on center of each chicken breast half. Fold long sides of chicken over chives mixture; fold up ends and secure with toothpick.

Mix cornflakes, parsley and paprika. Dip chicken into buttermilk, then lightly and evenly coat with cornflake mixture. Place chicken, seam sides down, in pan. Bake uncovered about 35 minutes or until chicken is no longer pink in center.

1 Serving:		% Daily Value:	
Calories	190	Vitamin A	18%
Calories from fat	55	Vitamin C	6%
Fat, g	6	Calcium	2%
Saturated, g	2	Iron	8%
Cholesterol, mg	60	**Diet Exchanges:**	
Sodium, mg	230	1/2 starch/bread	
Carbohydrate, g	9	3 lean meat	
Dietary Fiber, g	0		
Protein, g	25		

Garlic Chicken Kiev

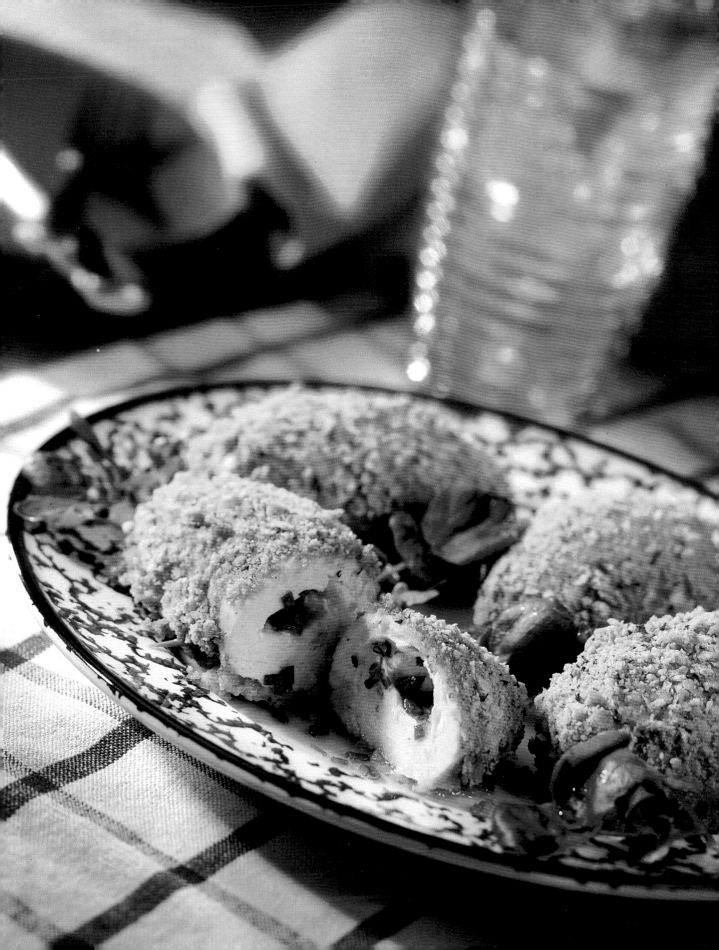

Chicken Breasts Dijon

PREP: 5 min; BAKE: 30 min

6 SERVINGS

6 skinless boneless chicken breast halves
    (1 1/2 pounds)

1/4 cup Dijon mustard

2 tablespoons dry white wine or chicken
    broth

Freshly ground pepper

2 tablespoons mustard seed

Heat oven to 400°. Spray rectangular pan, 13 × 9 × 2 inches, with nonstick cooking spray. Trim fat from chicken. Place chicken in pan. Mix mustard and wine; brush over chicken. Sprinkle with pepper and mustard seed. Bake uncovered about 30 minutes or until juice of chicken is no longer pink when centers of thickest pieces are cut.

1 Serving:		% Daily Value:	
Calories	155	Vitamin A	0%
Calories from fat	45	Vitamin C	0%
Fat, g	5	Calcium	2%
Saturated, g	1	Iron	8%
Cholesterol, mg	60	**Diet Exchanges:**	
Sodium, mg	190	3 lean meat	
Carbohydrate, g	1		
Dietary Fiber, g	0		
Protein, g	26		

Chicken with Fruit and Cheese

PREP: 5 min; COOK: 20 min

4 SERVINGS

4 skinless boneless chicken breast halves
    (1 pound)

1 tablespoon reduced-calorie spread

1 tablespoon water

1 jar (4 ounces) strained pears (baby food)

2/3 cup fresh or frozen cranberries

2 cups hot cooked brown rice

1 tablespoon sliced green onion

2 tablespoons crumbled feta cheese
    (1 ounce)

Trim fat from chicken. Melt spread in 10-inch nonstick skillet over medium-high heat. Cook chicken in spread, turning once, until brown. Add water to skillet. Spoon pears over chicken. Heat to boiling; reduce heat to low. Cover and simmer 10 minutes.

Sprinkle cranberries over chicken. Cover and simmer about 5 minutes or until juice of chicken is no longer pink when centers of thickest pieces are cut. Serve with rice. Sprinkle with onion and cheese.

1 Serving:		% Daily Value:	
Calories	265	Vitamin A	4%
Calories from fat	55	Vitamin C	8%
Fat, g	6	Calcium	4%
Saturated, g	2	Iron	8%
Cholesterol, mg	65	**Diet Exchanges:**	
Sodium, mg	150	1 starch/bread	
Carbohydrate, g	28	2 lean meat	
Dietary Fiber, g	3	1 fruit	
Protein, g	28		

RESTAURANT FOOD? YES!

If you've always enjoyed dining out but are reluctant because you're trying to lose weight, relax and make your reservations now!

Before Arriving at the Restaurant

- If you can, go to restaurants that offer healthier menu options or special low-fat entrées such as steamed vegetable plates (ask for it to be prepared without the butter). Or, look for menu descriptions that usually indicate cooking methods that are lower in fat such as broiled, roasted, grilled, poached or steamed. Avoid "all-you-can-eat" and fried-food establishments.

- Have in mind what you plan to order before arriving. You may even decide not to open the menu in order to avoid temptation.

- To avoid overeating, curb your appetite with a piece of fruit or large glass of water before you go.

At the Restaurant

Don't be afraid to ask that your food be prepared the way you want it; you're paying for it! Ask for:

- Information on how a dish is prepared; for example, are the steamed vegetables drizzled with butter? Are the roasted vegetables prepared with a lot of olive oil?

- Sauces and dressings on the side.

- Food prepared with no oil or butter; ask that it be cooked in wine or broth.

- An order to be split or ask for a half order.

- The server's help in removing tempting foods, such as having your plate taken away from the table so you won't continue to be tempted or eliminating a peek at the dessert tray.

Maple-Roasted Chicken with Wild Rice Stuffing

PREP: 10 min; COOK: 50 min

4 SERVINGS

Maple syrup basted onto boneless chicken breasts creates a sweet, fat-free glaze that complements the wild rice. Serve this roasted chicken with cranberry sauce for extra flavor.

3/4 cup ready-to-serve fat-free reduced-sodium chicken broth

1 medium onion, chopped (1/2 cup)

1 medium stalk celery, sliced (1/2 cup)

1/4 teaspoon poultry seasoning

1 cup herbed bread stuffing crumbs

1/2 cup cooked wild rice

4 skinless boneless chicken breast halves (1 pound)

3 tablespoons maple-flavored syrup

Heat oven to 375°. Spray square pan, 8 × 8 × 2 inches, with nonstick cooking spray. Heat 1/2 cup of the broth to boiling in 10-inch nonstick skillet. Cook onion, celery and poultry seasoning in broth 3 minutes, stirring frequently. Stir in stuffing crumbs and wild rice. Cook 1 minute; remove from heat. Stir in remaining 1/4 cup broth.

Trim fat from chicken. Flatten each chicken breast half to 1/4-inch thickness between waxed paper or plastic wrap. Divide stuffing mixture among chicken breast halves. Fold long sides of chicken over stuffing mixture; fold up ends and secure with toothpick.

Place chicken, seam sides down, in pan. Brush tops of chicken with maple syrup. Cover and bake about 45 minutes or until chicken is no longer pink in center.

1 Serving:		% Daily Value:	
Calories	225	Vitamin A	0%
Calories from fat	25	Vitamin C	2%
Fat, g	3	Calcium	2%
Saturated, g	1	Iron	8%
Cholesterol, mg	60	**Diet Exchanges:**	
Sodium, mg	220	1 starch/bread	
Carbohydrate, g	24	2 lean meat	
Dietary Fiber, g	1	2 vegetable	
Protein, g	27		

Southwestern Skillet Chicken and Couscous

PREP: 5 min; COOK: 19 min; STAND: 5 min

4 SERVINGS

4 skinless boneless chicken breast halves (1 pound)

1 1/2 cups ready-to-serve fat-free reduced-sodium chicken broth

1/2 teaspoon ground cumin

1/8 teaspoon pepper

1 cup uncooked couscous

1 can (7 ounces) whole kernel corn, drained

1 medium tomato, chopped (3/4 cup)

2 medium green onions, sliced (1/4 cup)

Spray 10-inch skillet with nonstick cooking spray; heat over medium heat. Cook chicken in skillet, turning once, until brown. Add 1/2 cup of the broth, the cumin and pepper. Heat to boiling; reduce heat to low. Cover and simmer about 7 minutes or until juice of chicken is no longer pink when centers of thickest pieces are cut.

Remove chicken from skillet with slotted spatula. Stir remaining 1 cup broth into skillet. Heat to boiling; remove from heat. Stir in couscous, corn, tomato and onions; place chicken on top. Cover and let stand 5 minutes.

1 Serving:		% Daily Value:	
Calories	320	Vitamin A	2%
Calories from fat	25	Vitamin C	8%
Fat, g	3	Calcium	4%
Saturated, g	1	Iron	12%
Cholesterol, mg	60	**Diet Exchanges:**	
Sodium, mg	340	3 starch/bread	
Carbohydrate, g	44	2 1/2 lean meat	
Dietary Fiber, g	3		
Protein, g	32		

Super-Easy Chicken Stir-Fry

PREP: 5 min; COOK: 9 min

4 SERVINGS

Just because you're busy, doesn't mean that you can't cook a healthful, satisfying meal! This stir-fry is so fast, it almost cooks itself.

1 pound skinless boneless chicken breast halves, cut into 1-inch pieces

1 package (16 ounces) frozen carrots, cauliflower and pea pods, thawed

1 clove garlic, finely chopped

1/2 cup stir-fry sauce

Hot cooked vermicelli or rice, if desired

Spray wok or 10-inch skillet with nonstick cooking spray; heat over medium-high heat. Add chicken; stir-fry about 5 minutes or until no longer pink in center.

Add vegetable mixture and garlic; stir-fry about 2 minutes or until vegetables are crisp-tender. Add stir-fry sauce. Cook and stir about 2 minutes or until heated through. Serve with vermicelli.

1 Serving:		% Daily Value:	
Calories	190	Vitamin A	36%
Calories from fat	45	Vitamin C	30%
Fat, g	5	Calcium	4%
Saturated, g	1	Iron	8%
Cholesterol, mg	60	**Diet Exchanges:**	
Sodium, mg	710	2 1/2 lean meat	
Carbohydrate, g	12	2 vegetable	
Dietary Fiber, g	3		
Protein, g	27		

Ginger Chicken with Curried Couscous

PREP: 5 min; MARINATE: 20 min; COOK: 15 min;
BROIL: 8 min

4 SERVINGS

1 tablespoon reduced-sodium soy sauce

1 tablespoon honey

1 tablespoon grated gingerroot

4 skinless boneless chicken breast halves
(1 pound)

2 1/4 cups ready-to-serve fat-free reduced-
sodium chicken broth

1 1/4 cups uncooked couscous

4 medium green onions, sliced (1/4 cup)

3/4 teaspoon curry powder

Mix soy sauce, honey and gingerroot in shallow
nonmetal dish or heavy-duty resealable plastic bag.
Add chicken; turn to coat. Cover dish or seal bag
and let stand 20 minutes at room temperature.

Heat broth to boiling in 10-inch nonstick skillet.
Stir in couscous, onions and curry powder; remove
from heat. Cover and let stand 8 to 10 minutes or
until broth is absorbed.

Meanwhile, set oven control to broil. Place chicken
on rack in broiler pan. Broil with tops 1 inch from
heat 5 minutes; turn. Broil about 3 minutes longer
or until juice is no longer pink when centers of
thickest pieces are cut. Serve over couscous.

1 Serving:		% Daily Value:	
Calories	360	Vitamin A	0%
Calories from fat	35	Vitamin C	2%
Fat, g	4	Calcium	4%
Saturated, g	1	Iron	12%
Cholesterol, mg	60	**Diet Exchanges:**	
Sodium, mg	460	3 starch/bread	
Carbohydrate, g	51	2 lean meat	
Dietary Fiber, g	3	1 vegetable	
Protein, g	33		

Chicken Niçoise

PREP: 10 min; COOK: 25 min

4 SERVINGS

*A small amount of olives and a bouquet of herbs lend
exotic flavor to this traditional dish from Nice,
France. Usually made with tuna fish, our chicken
version puts a new spin on an old classic.*

1 1/4 cups dry white wine or ready-to-serve
fat-free reduced-sodium chicken broth

4 skinless boneless chicken thighs or breasts
(1 pound)

3 cloves garlic, finely chopped

1/2 cup frozen pearl onions

1 tablespoon Italian seasoning

2 medium bell peppers, sliced

6 chopped pitted Kalamata olives (2 ounces)

2 cups hot cooked rice

Heat 1/4 cup of the wine to boiling in 10-inch
nonstick skillet. Cook chicken in wine, turning
once, until brown. Remove chicken from skillet;
keep warm.

Add garlic, onions, Italian seasoning, bell peppers,
olives and remaining 1 cup wine to skillet. Heat to
boiling; boil 5 minutes. Add chicken; reduce heat
to medium. Cook 10 to 15 minutes or until juice
of chicken is no longer pink when centers of thickest pieces are cut. Serve over rice.

1 Serving:		% Daily Value:	
Calories	290	Vitamin A	4%
Calories from fat	70	Vitamin C	28%
Fat, g	8	Calcium	6%
Saturated, g	3	Iron	20%
Cholesterol, mg	75	**Diet Exchanges:**	
Sodium, mg	130	2 starch/bread	
Carbohydrate, g	28	2 1/2 lean meat	
Dietary Fiber, g	1		
Protein, g	27		

Chicken Niçoise

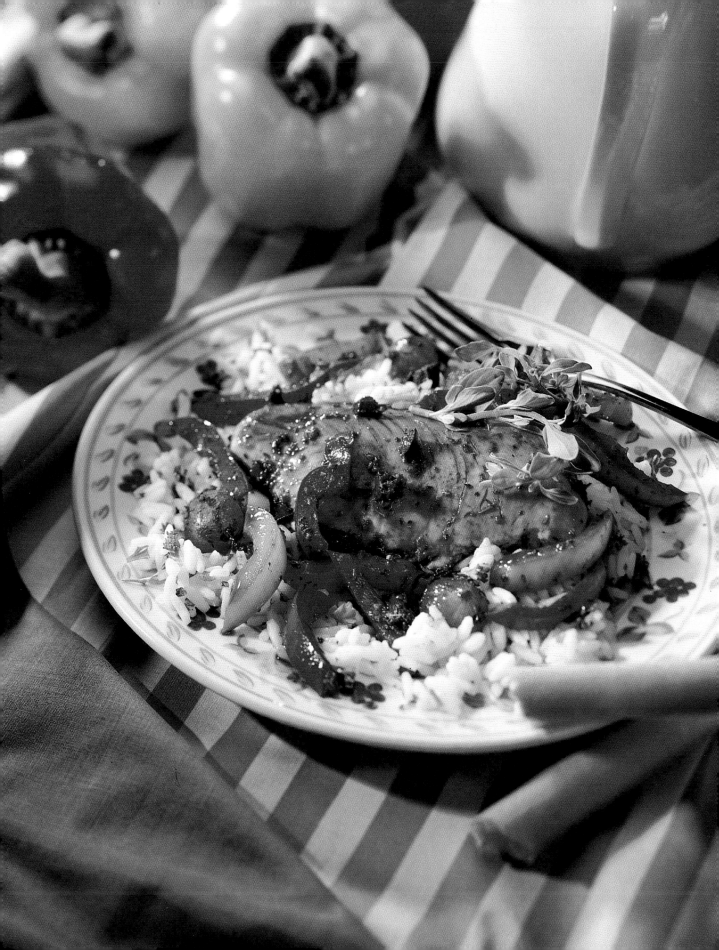

Oven-Fried Chicken Nuggets

PREP: 15 min; STAND: 5 min; BAKE: 30 min

6 SERVINGS

Fast food without the fat! You won't believe these tasty morsels that are baked in a cornflake-crumb crust.

2 pounds skinless boneless chicken breast halves

3/4 cup cornflakes

1/2 cup all-purpose flour

1 teaspoon paprika

3/4 teaspoon salt

1/2 teaspoon pepper

1/3 cup low-fat buttermilk

1/2 cup barbecue sauce

1/2 cup sweet-and-sour sauce

Heat oven to 400°. Line jelly roll pan, 15 1/2 × 10 1/2 × 1 inch, with aluminum foil. Trim fat from chicken. Cut chicken into 2-inch pieces. Place cornflakes, flour, paprika, salt and pepper in blender. Cover and blend on medium speed until cornflakes are reduced to crumbs; pour into bowl.

Place chicken and buttermilk in heavy resealable plastic bag; seal bag and let stand 5 minutes, turning once. Dip chicken into cornflake mixture to coat. Place in pan. Spray chicken with nonstick cooking spray.

Bake about 30 minutes or until crisp and chicken is no longer pink in center. Serve with barbecue sauce and sweet-and-sour sauce.

1 Serving:		% Daily Value:	
Calories	265	Vitamin A	6%
Calories from fat	45	Vitamin C	2%
Fat, g	5	Calcium	4%
Saturated, g	1	Iron	12%
Cholesterol, mg	85	**Diet Exchanges:**	
Sodium, mg	630	1 1/2 starch/bread	
Carbohydrate, g	21	3 lean meat	
Dietary Fiber, g	1		
Protein, g	35		

Oven-Fried Chicken Nuggets

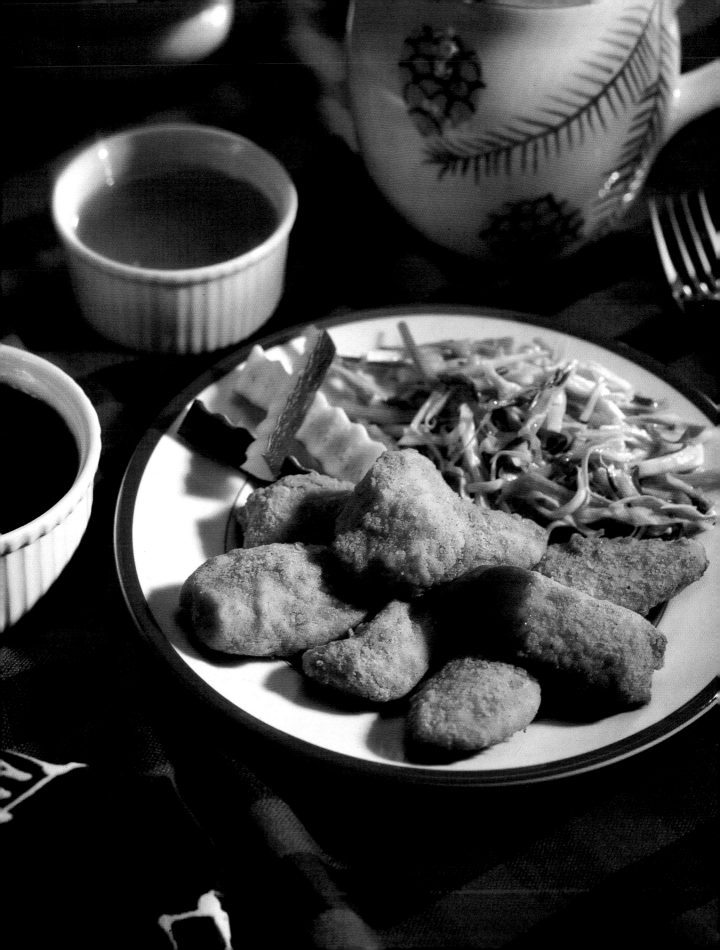

Savory Chicken and Rice

PREP: 5 min; COOK: 26 min

4 SERVINGS

1 pound skinless boneless chicken breast halves, cut into 1-inch pieces

1 1/2 cups sliced mushrooms (4 ounces)

1 cup baby-cut carrots

1 2/3 cups water

1 package (4.5 ounces) long grain and wild rice mix with almonds, chicken broth and herbs

Spray 10-inch skillet with nonstick cooking spray; heat over medium heat. Cook chicken in skillet about 5 minutes, stirring occasionally, until no longer pink in center. Stir in remaining ingredients.

Heat to boiling; reduce heat to low. Cover and simmer 15 minutes, stirring occasionally. Uncover and simmer about 3 minutes longer, stirring occasionally, until carrots are tender and liquid is absorbed.

1 Serving:		% Daily Value:	
Calories	290	Vitamin A	46%
Calories from fat	35	Vitamin C	2%
Fat, g	4	Calcium	4%
Saturated, g	1	Iron	14%
Cholesterol, mg	65	**Diet Exchanges:**	
Sodium, mg	700	2 starch/bread	
Carbohydrate, g	35	2 lean meat	
Dietary Fiber, g	2	1 vegetable	
Protein, g	30		

BEST MENU CHOICES

There are so many choices when dining out. To help you choose, we've listed some of the best menu options to select if you're trying to watch what you're eating.

Appetizers: Shrimp cocktail, broth-based or bean soups, grilled or roasted vegetables (without oil), grilled polenta without cheese, salad with low-fat or fat-free dressing or dressing on the side, and bread without butter or olive oil.

Seafood: Choose broiled, grilled or poached. Good choices include salmon, swordfish, flounder, whitefish, halibut, grouper, orange roughy, walleye, shrimp, scallops and lobster. Season fish with fresh lemon, cocktail sauce or horseradish rather than melted butter or tartar sauce.

Italian: Choose tomato sauces versus cream sauce or pesto. Meatless tomato sauces are usually available. Order plain pasta rather than cheese- or meat-filled ravioli, tortellini and stuffed manicotti. Skip the butter or olive oil and Parmesan cheese with your bread. Avoid dishes with a lot of cheese or ask that if cheese is used for a topping, that it be left off, or half the amount used.

Chinese: Choose chow mein, lo-mein, vegetable mixtures with chicken, seafood, beef or pork, meatless stir-fries, steamed dishes and white rice. Ask that no oil be used to prepare your food.

Mexican: Choose fajitas and ask that no oil be used to cook the meat or chicken and onions and peppers. Other choices might be soft tacos with beef or chicken, black bean or chicken burritos and chicken enchiladas without the cheese. When ordering, ask that sides of cheese and guacamole not be brought to the table and unless they offer low-fat or fat-free sour cream, skip that too and request extra salsa instead. Avoid snacking on the predinner chips and salsa unless the chips are baked and not fried or sample a cup of broth-based soup or meatless chili.

Japanese: Choose grilled, broiled, simmered and steamed entrees such as teriyaki, yosenabe or shabu-shabu. Plain white rice is a good choice to go with your meal but remember that one cup has 200 calories.

Dessert: If you only want a couple of bites of rich dessert, share it with it with your companions or choose low-fat frozen yogurt, sorbets, ices, fresh fruit or order coffee, tea or an espresso drink (made with low-fat milk) instead of a traditional dessert.

Chicken Fricassee with Mushrooms

PREP: 5 min; COOK: 30 min

4 SERVINGS

A small amount of fat-free sour cream goes a long way in this southern dish, which is short on calories and fat.

2 teaspoons olive or vegetable oil

4 skinless boneless chicken thighs (1 pound)

1/3 cup ready-to-serve fat-free reduced-sodium chicken broth

2 cups sliced mushrooms (6 ounces)

1 cup frozen carrots, onions and red peppers (from 16-ounce package)

1 can (14 1/2 ounces) whole tomatoes, undrained

1/4 cup fat-free sour cream

1/2 teaspoon salt

Heat oil in 10-inch nonstick skillet over medium-high heat. Cook chicken in oil, turning once, until brown.

Stir in broth, mushrooms, vegetable mixture and tomatoes, breaking up tomatoes. Heat to boiling; reduce heat to low. Simmer uncovered about 15 minutes or until juice of chicken is no longer pink when centers of thickest pieces are cut. Remove chicken from skillet; keep warm.

Cook vegetable mixture in skillet over high heat about 5 minutes, stirring occasionally, until thickened; remove from heat. Stir in sour cream and salt. Serve vegetable mixture over chicken.

1 Serving:		% Daily Value:	
Calories	215	Vitamin A	12%
Calories from fat	80	Vitamin C	18%
Fat, g	9	Calcium	8%
Saturated, g	2	Iron	16%
Cholesterol, mg	75	**Diet Exchanges:**	
Sodium, mg	650	3 lean meat	
Carbohydrate, g	9	2 vegetable	
Dietary Fiber, g	2		
Protein, g	27		

Grilled Chicken Drumsticks

PREP: 10 min; GRILL: 1 hr

4 SERVINGS

**8 chicken drumsticks or thighs
   (1 1/2 pounds)**

2 tablespoons soy sauce

1 tablespoon olive or vegetable oil

1 teaspoon Dijon mustard

1/4 teaspoon salt

1/8 teaspoon ground red pepper (cayenne)

2 cloves garlic, finely chopped

Chopped fresh cilantro, if desired

Heat coals or gas grill for direct heat. Remove skin and fat from chicken. Mix remaining ingredients except cilantro; brush over chicken. Cover and grill chicken, bone sides down, 4 to 6 inches from medium heat 15 to 20 minutes; turn. Cover and grill 20 to 40 minutes longer, turning 2 or 3 times, until juice of chicken is no longer pink when centers of thickest pieces are cut. Sprinkle with cilantro.

Broiling Directions: Set oven control to broil. Place chicken, skin sides down, on rack in broiler pan. Brush with oil mixture. Broil chicken with tops 7 to 9 inches from heat 20 minutes; turn. Brush with oil mixture. Broil 10 to 15 minutes longer or until juice of chicken is no longer pink when centers of thickest pieces are cut.

1 Serving:		% Daily Value:	
Calories	175	Vitamin A	0%
Calories from fat	65	Vitamin C	0%
Fat, g	7	Calcium	2%
Saturated, g	2	Iron	6%
Cholesterol, mg	70	**Diet Exchanges:**	
Sodium, mg	740	3 lean meat	
Carbohydrate, g	1		
Dietary Fiber, g	0		
Protein, g	27		

Southwestern Chicken and White Bean Chili

PREP: 10 min; COOK: 26 min

4 SERVINGS

Jalapeño chilies and chili powder give depth and spiciness to this quick-cooking meal-in-a-bowl. Top with chopped cilantro and crushed baked tortilla chips for extra zip.

1/2 cup ready-to-serve fat-free reduced-sodium chicken broth

2 skinless boneless chicken thighs (1/2 pound), diced

2 cups frozen carrots, onions and green beans (from 16-ounce package)

2 teaspoons chili powder

1 teaspoon chopped fresh or canned jalapeño chilies

1 can (15 to 16 ounces) cannellini or great northern beans, undrained

1 can (16 ounces) stewed tomatoes, undrained

1/4 cup reduced-fat sour cream

Heat broth to boiling in Dutch oven. Cook chicken in broth, stirring occasionally, until brown. Stir in remaining ingredients except sour cream. Heat to boiling; reduce heat to medium-high. Cover and cook about 20 minutes or until thickened. Top each serving with sour cream.

1 Serving:		% Daily Value:	
Calories	265	Vitamin A	16%
Calories from fat	45	Vitamin C	16%
Fat, g	5	Calcium	18%
Saturated, g	1	Iron	34%
Cholesterol, mg	45	**Diet Exchanges:**	
Sodium, mg	560	2 starch/bread	
Carbohydrate, g	39	1 lean meat	
Dietary Fiber, g	10	2 vegetable	
Protein, g	26		

Turkey-Pasta Primavera

PREP: 5 min; COOK: 9 min

4 SERVINGS

2 tablespoons fat-free Italian dressing

1 package (16 ounces) frozen broccoli, cauliflower and carrots, thawed

2 cups cut-up cooked turkey or chicken breast

1 teaspoon salt

2 large tomatoes, seeded and chopped (2 cups)

4 cups hot cooked spaghetti or fettuccine

1/4 cup freshly grated Parmesan cheese (1 ounce)

2 tablespoons chopped fresh parsley

Heat dressing in 10-inch skillet over medium-high heat. Cook vegetable mixture in dressing, stirring occasionally, until vegetables are crisp-tender. Stir in turkey, salt and tomatoes. Cook about 3 minutes or just until turkey is hot. Spoon turkey mixture over spaghetti. Sprinkle with cheese and parsley.

1 Serving:		% Daily Value:	
Calories	345	Vitamin A	42%
Calories from fat	65	Vitamin C	42%
Fat, g	7	Calcium	14%
Saturated, g	2	Iron	22%
Cholesterol, mg	60	**Diet Exchanges:**	
Sodium, mg	820	3 starch/bread	
Carbohydrate, g	49	2 lean meat	
Dietary Fiber, g	5	1 vegetable	
Protein, g	31		

Turkey Pie

PREP: 5 min; BAKE: 35 min; STAND: 5 min

6 SERVINGS

This easy turkey pie makes its own crust!

2 cups cut-up cooked turkey or chicken breast

1 jar (4 1/2 ounces) sliced mushrooms, drained

4 medium green onions, sliced (1/2 cup)

1 cup shredded reduced-fat Swiss cheese (4 ounces)

3/4 cup Bisquick Reduced Fat baking mix

1 1/3 cups skim milk

1 cup fat-free cholesterol-free egg product or 2 eggs plus 2 egg whites

Heat oven to 400°. Spray pie plate, 10 × 1 1/2 inches, with nonstick cooking spray. Sprinkle turkey, mushrooms, onions and cheese in pie plate. Stir remaining ingredients with fork until blended. Pour into pie plate.

Bake 30 to 35 minutes or until golden brown and knife inserted halfway between center and edge comes out clean. Let stand 5 minutes before cutting.

1 Serving:		% Daily Value:	
Calories	225	Vitamin A	6%
Calories from fat	65	Vitamin C	0%
Fat, g	7	Calcium	34%
Saturated, g	3	Iron	12%
Cholesterol, mg	45	**Diet Exchanges:**	
Sodium, mg	380	1 starch/bread	
Carbohydrate, g	15	2 1/2 lean meat	
Dietary Fiber, g	1		
Protein, g	26		

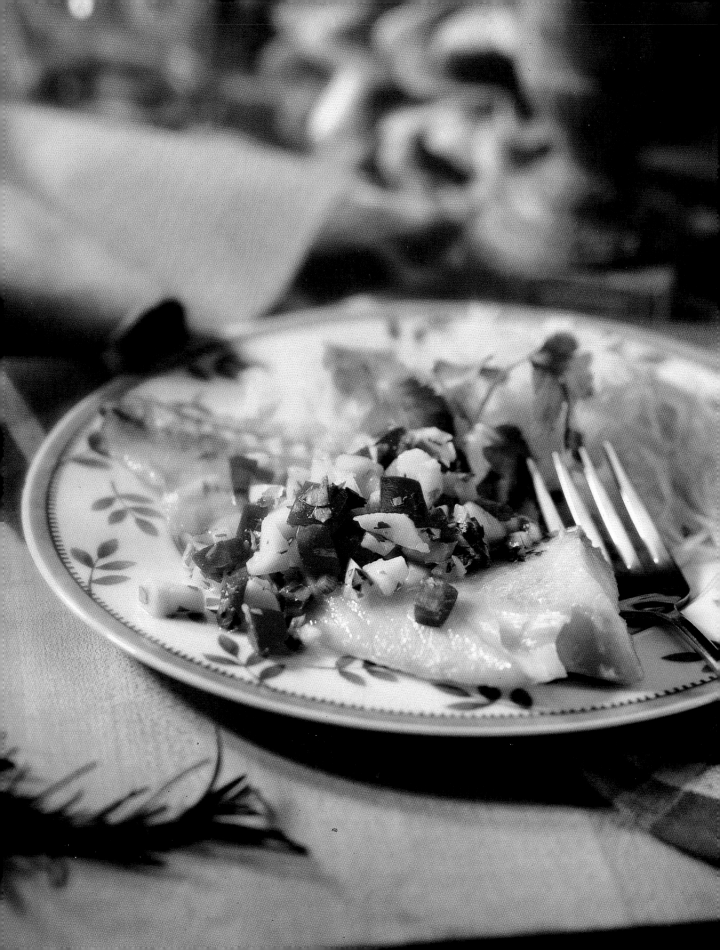

5

Fabulous Fish and Seafood

Red Snapper with Tropical Relish
(page 114)

Crunchy Baked Fish

PREP: 10 min; BAKE: 15 min

4 SERVINGS

1 pound flounder, sole or orange roughy fillets

1/3 cup finely crushed reduced-fat cheese crackers

1 teaspoon dried parsley flakes

3 tablespoons fat-free Western or French dressing

Heat oven to 450°. Spray cookie sheet with nonstick cooking spray. If fish fillets are large, cut into 4 serving pieces. Mix crackers and parsley. Brush both sides of fish with dressing; coat one side of fish with cracker mixture. Place fish, cracker sides up, on cookie sheet. Bake uncovered 10 to 15 minutes or until fish flakes easily with fork.

1 Serving:		% Daily Value:	
Calories	145	Vitamin A	0%
Calories from fat	35	Vitamin C	0%
Fat, g	4	Calcium	2%
Saturated, g	1	Iron	2%
Cholesterol, mg	55	**Diet Exchanges:**	
Sodium, mg	290	1/2 starch/bread	
Carbohydrate, g	8	2 lean meat	
Dietary Fiber, g	1		
Protein, g	20		

Crispy Baked Catfish

PREP: 10 min; BAKE: 18 min

4 SERVINGS

1/4 cup yellow cornmeal

1/4 cup dry bread crumbs

1 teaspoon chili powder

1/2 teaspoon paprika

1/2 teaspoon garlic salt

1/4 teaspoon pepper

1 pound catfish fillets

1/4 cup fat-free French or ranch dressing

Heat oven to 450°. Spray broiler pan rack with nonstick cooking spray. Mix cornmeal, bread crumbs, chili powder, paprika, garlic salt and pepper.

If fish fillets are large, cut into 4 serving pieces. Lightly brush dressing on all sides of fish. Coat fish with cornmeal mixture. Place fish on rack in broiler pan. Bake uncovered 15 to 18 minutes or until fish flakes easily with fork.

1 Serving:		% Daily Value:	
Calories	180	Vitamin A	4%
Calories from fat	20	Vitamin C	0%
Fat, g	2	Calcium	4%
Saturated, g	0	Iron	8%
Cholesterol, mg	70	**Diet Exchanges:**	
Sodium, mg	510	1 starch/bread	
Carbohydrate, g	15	2 lean meat	
Dietary Fiber, g	1		
Protein, g	26		

Crispy Baked Catfish

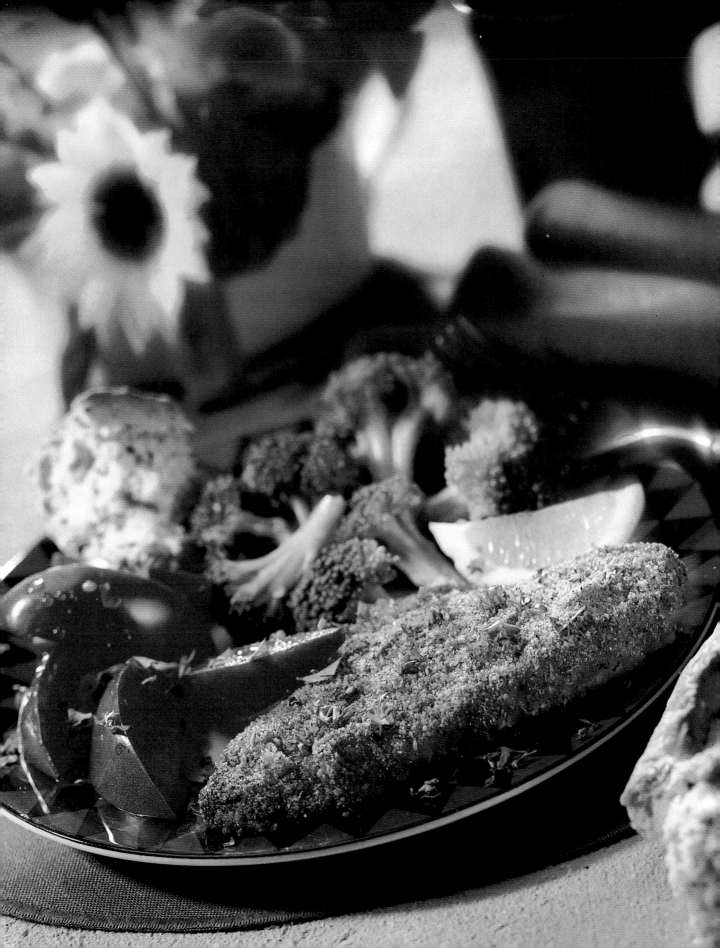

Oven-Fried Fish Fillets with Tangy Maple Sauce

PREP: 5 min; COOK: 20 min

4 SERVINGS

1 pound walleye or orange roughy fillets

1/3 cup fat-free buttermilk

3/4 cup cornflakes, crushed

1/2 cup all-purpose flour

1/4 teaspoon salt

1/4 teaspoon freshly ground pepper

1/2 cup barbecue sauce

2 tablespoons maple-flavored syrup

Heat oven to 400°. Line jelly roll pan, 15 1/2 × 1 1/2 × 1 inch, with aluminum foil. Spray foil with nonstick cooking spray.

Place fish and buttermilk in heavy-duty resealable plastic bag. Seal bag and shake well to coat fish. Mix cornflakes, flour, salt and pepper. Coat fish with cornflake mixture. Place fish in pan. Spray fish with nonstick cooking spray.

Bake uncovered 15 to 20 minutes or until fish is light brown and flakes easily with fork. Mix barbecue sauce and maple syrup. Serve sauce with fish.

1 Serving:		% Daily Value:	
Calories	230	Vitamin A	8%
Calories from fat	20	Vitamin C	4%
Fat, g	2	Calcium	4%
Saturated, g	0	Iron	8%
Cholesterol, mg	65	**Diet Exchanges:**	
Sodium, mg	570	1 starch/bread	
Carbohydrate, g	29	2 lean meat	
Dietary Fiber, g	1	1 fruit	
Protein, g	25		

Red Snapper with Tropical Relish

PREP: 10 min; MARINATE: 30 min; BROIL: 8 min

4 SERVINGS

Refreshing tropical fruit flavors top this lightly broiled or grilled fish. Mangoes vary in sweetness, so start with the lesser amount of lime juice and add more as desired.

1 large mango, papaya or peach, seeded, peeled and diced (3/4 cup)

1 small tomato, diced (1/2 cup)

1/2 cup chopped fresh cilantro

2 tablespoons finely chopped red onion

1/4 cup lime juice

1 pound red snapper, orange roughy or walleye fillets

1/2 teaspoon salt

Mix mango, tomato, onion, cilantro and lime juice in nonmetal bowl. Cover and let stand 30 minutes.

Set oven control to broil. Place fish on rack in broiler pan. Spray fish with nonstick cooking spray; sprinkle with salt. Broil with tops 4 to 6 inches from heat 5 to 8 minutes or until fish is light brown and flakes easily with fork. Serve with relish.

1 Serving:		% Daily Value:	
Calories	150	Vitamin A	22%
Calories from fat	20	Vitamin C	20%
Fat, g	2	Calcium	2%
Saturated, g	1	Iron	2%
Cholesterol, mg	60	**Diet Exchanges:**	
Sodium, mg	390	2 lean meat	
Carbohydrate, g	12	1 vegetable	
Dietary Fiber, g	1	1/2 fruit	
Protein, g	22		

Baked Salmon with Persimmon Salsa

PREP: 8 min; BAKE: 20 min

4 SERVINGS

Bright and tangy persimmon is a colorful topping for this baked fish, and is especially nice in winter weather. Choose a persimmon that is completely soft and bright in color for the sweetest flavor.

1 pound salmon fillets

1/4 cup lemon juice

1 1/2 cups chopped peeled persimmons or pears

1/4 cup chopped fresh cilantro

1 teaspoon chopped fresh or canned jalapeño chilies

Heat oven to 400°. Place fish in ungreased rectangular baking dish, 11 × 7 × 1 1/2. Drizzle 2 tablespoons of the lemon juice over fish.

Bake uncovered 15 to 20 minutes or until fish flakes easily with fork. Mix remaining 2 tablespoons lemon juice and remaining ingredients. Serve persimmon mixture over fish.

1 Serving:		% Daily Value:	
Calories	195	Vitamin A	16%
Calories from fat	65	Vitamin C	8%
Fat, g	7	Calcium	2%
Saturated, g	2	Iron	4%
Cholesterol, mg	75	**Diet Exchanges:**	
Sodium, mg	70	3 lean meat	
Carbohydrate, g	11	1/2 fruit	
Dietary Fiber, g	2		
Protein, g	24		

Salmon Teriyaki

PREP: 5 min; MARINATE: 1 hr; BROIL: 7 min

2 SERVINGS

2 tablespoons reduced-sodium soy sauce

3 tablespoons dry white wine or orange juice

1/4 cup packed brown sugar

1/2 teaspoon ground ginger or 1 teaspoon grated gingerroot

1/2 pound salmon fillets

Mix soy sauce, wine, brown sugar and ginger in shallow nonmetal dish. Add fish, turning several times to coat with marinade. Cover and refrigerate 1 hour, turning once.

Set oven control to broil. Spray broiler pan rack with nonstick cooking spray. Remove fish from marinade; reserve marinade. Place fish on rack in broiler pan. Broil with tops 4 to 6 inches from heat 5 to 6 minutes or until fish flakes easily with fork. Heat marinade to boiling; boil and stir 1 minute. Serve marinade with fish.

1 Serving:		% Daily Value:	
Calories	205	Vitamin A	2%
Calories from fat	55	Vitamin C	0%
Fat, g	6	Calcium	2%
Saturated, g	2	Iron	6%
Cholesterol, mg	75	**Diet Exchanges:**	
Sodium, mg	370	3 lean meat	
Carbohydrate, g	14	1 fruit	
Dietary Fiber, g	0		
Protein, g	24		

Halibut with Lime and Cilantro

PREP: 10 min; MARINATE: 1 hr; BROIL: 12 min

2 SERVINGS

2 tablespoons lime juice

1 tablespoon chopped cilantro

1 teaspoon olive or vegetable oil

1 clove garlic, finely chopped

2 halibut or salmon steaks (about 3/4 pound)

Freshly ground pepper to taste

1/2 cup salsa

Mix lime juice, cilantro, oil and garlic in rectangular pan, 11 × 7 × 1 1/2 inches. Add fish, turning several times to coat with marinade. Cover and refrigerate 1 hour, turning once.

Set oven control to broil. Spray broiler pan rack with nonstick cooking spray. Remove fish from marinade; discard marinade. Place fish on rack in broiler pan. Broil with tops 4 inches from heat 8 to 12 minutes, turning once, until fish flakes easily with fork. Sprinkle with pepper. Serve with salsa.

1 Serving:		% Daily Value:	
Calories	185	Vitamin A	6%
Calories from fat	35	Vitamin C	14%
Fat, g	4	Calcium	6%
Saturated, g	1	Iron	6%
Cholesterol, mg	90	**Diet Exchanges:**	
Sodium, mg	310	3 lean meat	
Carbohydrate, g	5	1 vegetable	
Dietary Fiber, g	1		
Protein, g	33		

Mediterranean Halibut

PREP: 10 min; CHILL: 1 hr; BAKE: 30 min

4 SERVINGS

1 pound halibut, cod or red snapper fillets

2 tablespoons lemon juice

1 tablespoon chopped onion

1 tablespoon chopped pimiento

1 tablespoon coarsely chopped pimiento-stuffed olives

1 tablespoon capers

1 tablespoon olive or vegetable oil

If fish fillets are large, cut into 4 serving pieces. Place fish in ungreased square baking dish, 8 × 8 × 2 inches. Mix remaining ingredients; spread over fish. Cover and refrigerate at least 1 hour, turning once.

Heat oven to 350°. Cover and bake 20 to 30 minutes or until fish flakes easily with fork.

1 Serving:		% Daily Value:	
Calories	115	Vitamin A	0%
Calories from fat	25	Vitamin C	2%
Fat, g	3	Calcium	2%
Saturated, g	1	Iron	2%
Cholesterol, mg	60	**Diet Exchanges:**	
Sodium, mg	150	2 lean meat	
Carbohydrate, g	1		
Dietary Fiber, g	0		
Protein, g	21		

Broiled Walleye with Tomato-Caper Sauce

PREP: 5 min; COOK: 20 min; BROIL: 5 min

4 SERVINGS

Use any firm fish, such as tuna, swordfish or salmon, for this savory dish.

1 can (28 ounces) whole tomatoes, drained and juice reserved

1 large onion, thinly sliced

3 cloves garlic, finely chopped

2 tablespoons capers

1 pound walleye, orange roughy or red snapper fillets

Heat reserved tomato juice to boiling in 10-inch nonstick skillet; reduce heat to medium. Stir in onion, garlic and capers. Cook 3 minutes. Stir in tomatoes, breaking up tomatoes. Cover and cook about 15 minutes or until sauce is thickened.

Set oven control to broil. Place fish on rack in broiler pan. Spray fish with nonstick cooking spray. Broil with tops 4 to 6 inches from heat 3 to 5 minutes or until fish is light brown and flakes easily with fork. Serve sauce over fish.

1 Serving:		% Daily Value:	
Calories	155	Vitamin A	12%
Calories from fat	20	Vitamin C	26%
Fat, g	2	Calcium	8%
Saturated, g	0	Iron	8%
Cholesterol, mg	60	**Diet Exchanges:**	
Sodium, mg	530	2 lean meat	
Carbohydrate, g	13	2 vegetable	
Dietary Fiber, g	3		
Protein, g	24		

Fish with Summer Vegetables

PREP: 10 min; BAKE: 30 min

4 SERVINGS

1 pound cod, halibut or red snapper fillets

1 tablespoon lemon juice

Freshly ground pepper

1 small zucchini or yellow summer squash, thinly sliced (1 cup)

1 small onion, thinly sliced

1 tablespoon chopped fresh or 1 teaspoon dried basil leaves

1 can (8 ounces) stewed tomatoes, undrained

2 tablespoons grated Parmesan cheese

Heat oven to 350°. If fish fillets are large, cut into 4 serving pieces. Place fish in ungreased rectangular baking dish, 11 × 7 × 1 1/2 inches. Sprinkle with lemon juice and pepper. Layer zucchini and onion on fish. Sprinkle with basil; top with tomatoes. Cover and bake 20 to 30 minutes or until fish flakes easily with fork. Sprinkle with cheese.

1 Serving:		% Daily Value:	
Calories	135	Vitamin A	6%
Calories from fat	20	Vitamin C	12%
Fat, g	2	Calcium	8%
Saturated, g	1	Iron	4%
Cholesterol, mg	60	**Diet Exchanges:**	
Sodium, mg	230	2 lean meat	
Carbohydrate, g	6	1 vegetable	
Dietary Fiber, g	1		
Protein, g	24		

Louisiana Seafood Creole

PREP: 5 min; COOK: 35 min
4 SERVINGS

Packaged frozen vegetables and canned tomatoes make this flavorful supper dish a snap.

1/2 cup dry white wine or ready-to-serve fat-free reduced-sodium chicken broth

3 cups frozen green beans, red peppers and carrots (from 16-ounce package)

4 large cloves garlic, finely chopped (1 tablespoon)

1/4 to 1/2 teaspoon ground red pepper (cayenne)

1/2 pound cod, halibut or red snapper fillets, cubed

1 can (16 ounces) stewed tomatoes, undrained

1 pound uncooked, peeled, deveined small shrimp, thawed if frozen

Hot cooked rice, if desired

Heat 1/4 cup of the wine to boiling in 4-quart Dutch oven or saucepan. Stir in vegetable mixture and garlic. Cook about 10 minutes, stirring frequently, until liquid has evaporated. Stir in remaining wine, the red pepper, fish and tomatoes. Heat to boiling; reduce heat to medium. Cover and cook 20 minutes.

Stir in shrimp. Cook about 5 to 7 minutes or until shrimp are pink and firm. Serve over rice.

1 Serving:		% Daily Value:	
Calories	175	Vitamin A	74%
Calories from fat	20	Vitamin C	58%
Fat, g	2	Calcium	10%
Saturated, g	1	Iron	22%
Cholesterol, mg	190	**Diet Exchanges:**	
Sodium, mg	420	2 lean meat	
Carbohydrate, g	12	2 vegetable	
Dietary Fiber, g	3		
Protein, g	30		

Orange Roughy with Red Peppers

PREP: 10 min; COOK: 30 min
4 SERVINGS

1 pound orange roughy, walleye or sole fillets

1 teaspoon olive or vegetable oil

1 small onion, cut into thin slices

2 medium red bell peppers, cut into julienne strips

1 tablespoon chopped fresh or 1 teaspoon dried thyme leaves

1/2 teaspoon salt

1/4 teaspoon pepper

If fish fillets are large, cut into 4 serving pieces. Heat oil in 10-inch nonstick skillet over medium heat. Layer onion and bell peppers in skillet. Sprinkle with half of the thyme and pepper. Layer fish on bell peppers. Sprinkle with remaining thyme, salt and pepper. Reduce heat to medium. Cover and cook 15 minutes. Uncover and cook 5 to 10 minutes longer or until fish flakes easily with fork.

1 Serving:		% Daily Value:	
Calories	125	Vitamin A	4%
Calories from fat	25	Vitamin C	28%
Fat, g	3	Calcium	2%
Saturated, g	1	Iron	4%
Cholesterol, mg	60	**Diet Exchanges:**	
Sodium, mg	100	2 lean meat	
Carbohydrate, g	4	1 vegetable	
Dietary Fiber, g	1		
Protein, g	22		

Orange Roughy with Red Peppers

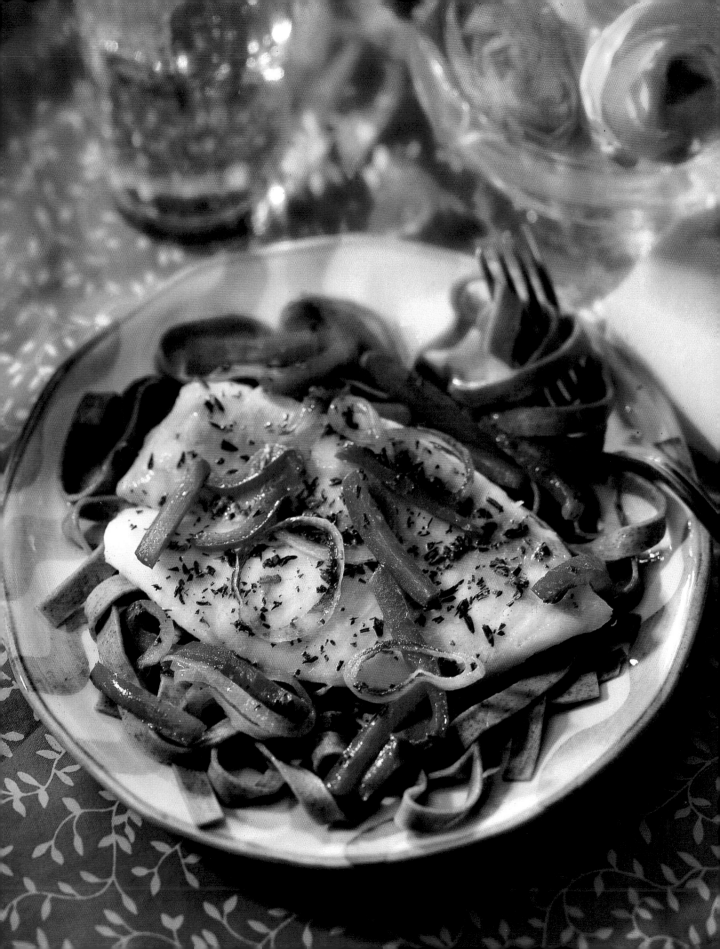

Lemon-Curry Cod

PREP: 5; BROIL: 8 min

4 SERVINGS

1 pound cod, halibut or red snapper fillets

1 tablespoon coconut, if desired

2 tablespoons reduced-fat mayonnaise or salad dressing

2 tablespoons honey

1 tablespoon lemon juice

1 tablespoon Dijon mustard

1 teaspoon curry powder

1/2 teaspoon salt

Set oven control to broil. Spray broiler pan rack with nonstick cooking spray. Place fish on rack in broiler pan. Mix remaining ingredients; spread evenly over fish. Broil with tops 4 to 6 inches from heat 5 to 8 minutes or until fish flakes easily with fork.

1 Serving:		% Daily Value:	
Calories	165	Vitamin A	0%
Calories from fat	35	Vitamin C	0%
Fat, g	4	Calcium	2%
Saturated, g	1	Iron	2%
Cholesterol, mg	60	**Diet Exchanges:**	
Sodium, mg	480	2 1/2 lean meat	
Carbohydrate, g	10	1/2 fruit	
Dietary Fiber, g	0		
Protein, g	22		

Thai Fish Stew

PREP: 5 min; COOK: 20 min

4 SERVINGS

Easy and fast, this sweet and spicy stew will warm the coldest winter evening. Oriental palm sugar lends an exotic hint of coconut flavor.

1/2 cup clam juice

4 cloves garlic, finely chopped

3 cups packaged fresh stir-fry vegetables

1/2 pound cod or halibut fillets, cubed

1 1/2 tablespoons chopped fresh or canned jalapeño chilies

2 tablespoons fish sauce or reduced-sodium soy sauce

1 tablespoon packed brown sugar or Oriental palm sugar

4 cups hot cooked rice

Heat 1/4 cup of the clam juice to boiling in 10-inch nonstick skillet. Cook garlic in clam juice 1 minute. Stir in stir-fry vegetables. Cook about 8 minutes, stirring frequently, until liquid has evaporated.

Stir in fish, chilies, fish sauce and brown sugar. Heat to boiling; reduce heat to medium. Simmer uncovered 10 minutes. Serve over rice.

1 Serving:		% Daily Value:	
Calories	305	Vitamin A	16%
Calories from fat	20	Vitamin C	32%
Fat, g	2	Calcium	6%
Saturated, g	0	Iron	18%
Cholesterol, mg	30	**Diet Exchanges:**	
Sodium, mg	780	2 starch/bread	
Carbohydrate, g	57	1 lean meat	
Dietary Fiber, g	3	2 vegetable	
Protein, g	18	1 fruit	

Scallops with Red Pepper Sauce

PREP: 5 min; COOK: 16 min

4 SERVINGS

1 large red bell pepper, cut into fourths

1/8 teaspoon salt

10 drops red pepper sauce

1 clove garlic, finely chopped

1/4 cup plain fat-free yogurt

1 pound bay scallops

3 medium green onions, sliced (1/3 cup)

Place steamer basket in 1/2 inch water in saucepan or skillet (water should not touch bottom of basket). Place bell pepper in basket. Cover tightly and heat to boiling; reduce heat. Steam 8 to 10 minutes or until tender.

Place bell pepper, salt, pepper sauce and garlic in blender or food processor. Cover and blend on medium speed until almost smooth. Heat red pepper mixture in 1-quart saucepan over medium heat, stirring occasionally, until hot; remove from heat. Gradually beat in yogurt, using wire whisk.

Spray 10-inch nonstick skillet with nonstick cooking spray; heat over medium-high heat. Add scallops and onions; stir-fry 4 to 5 minutes or until scallops are white. Serve scallops with sauce.

1 Serving:		% Daily Value:	
Calories	150	Vitamin A	20%
Calories from fat	20	Vitamin C	42%
Fat, g	2	Calcium	16%
Saturated, g	0	Iron	20%
Cholesterol, mg	35	**Diet Exchanges:**	
Sodium, mg	390	2 1/2 lean meat	
Carbohydrate, g	7	1 vegetable	
Dietary Fiber, g	1		
Protein, g	27		

ALL I NEED TO WORRY ABOUT IS FAT

Fact: Nutrition experts advise that each food we eat be less than 30 percent fat.

False: Recommendations by experts are to keep our *daily* intake under 30 percent of calories from fat out of total calories consumed, so it isn't necessary for every food to be that low. To calculate the percent of fat in a food, use the following formula (this example uses the recipe Pork, Onion and Pepper Fajitas on page 146):

1. Multiply total grams of fat per serving times 9 calories per gram of fat.

   Example: 3 g fat in recipe for each serving × 9 cal/g = 27 calories from the fat.

2. Divide 27 calories from fat by the total number of calories per serving in the recipe or product.

   Example: 27 calories from fat ÷ 220 = 0.12

3. Multiply the number you got from step 2 by 100.

   Example: 0.12 × 100 = 12% of calories are from fat

Fact: Simply cutting fat is all you need to do to lose weight.

False: Though eliminating excess fat from the diet is generally helpful in aiding people shed extra pounds, it doesn't work for everyone. Calories count too. And if you eat more calories than you burn, you won't lose weight. Getting regular exercise and changing behaviors that trigger overeating are important keys to successful weight loss.

Shrimp-Pesto Pasta

PREP: 5 min; MARINATE: 15 min; COOK: 5 min

4 SERVINGS

Prepared pesto thinned with fat-free yogurt slashes the fat, and keeps preparation simple. Serve with extra grated Parmesan cheese, if you like.

1/2 pound uncooked peeled deveined medium shrimp, thawed if frozen

2 tablespoons lemon juice

4 large cloves garlic, finely chopped (1 tablespoon)

1 teaspoon grated lemon peel

3 tablespoons pesto

1/4 cup plain fat-free yogurt

4 cups hot cooked spaghetti

Mix shrimp, lemon juice and garlic in shallow nonmetal dish or heavy-duty resealable plastic bag. Cover dish or seal bag and let stand 15 minutes at room temperature.

Spray 10-inch nonstick skillet with nonstick cooking spray; heat over medium-high heat. Cook shrimp mixture in skillet about 5 minutes, stirring occasionally, until lemon juice has evaporated. Mix lemon peel, pesto and yogurt; toss with spaghetti and shrimp.

1 Serving:		% Daily Value:	
Calories	315	Vitamin A	2%
Calories from fat	80	Vitamin C	4%
Fat, g	9	Calcium	10%
Saturated, g	2	Iron	20%
Cholesterol, mg	85	**Diet Exchanges:**	
Sodium, mg	150	3 starch/bread	
Carbohydrate, g	43	1 1/2 lean meat	
Dietary Fiber, g	2		
Protein, g	17		

Grilled Shrimp Kabobs

PREP: 10 min; MARINATE: 30 min; GRILL: 8 min

2 SERVINGS

1/2 pound uncooked, peeled, deveined large shrimp, thawed if frozen

1/2 cup fat-free Italian dressing

1/2 medium red onion, cut into 8 pieces

1/2 medium green bell pepper, cut into 8 pieces

8 medium cherry tomatoes

8 small whole mushrooms

2 cups hot cooked orzo pasta or rice

Place shrimp and dressing in shallow nonmetal dish or heavy-duty resealable plastic bag. Cover dish or seal bag and refrigerate 30 minutes.

Heat coals or gas grill for direct heat. Remove shrimp from marinade; reserve marinade. Thread shrimp, onion, bell pepper, tomatoes and mushrooms alternately on each of four 15-inch metal skewers, leaving space between each.

Grill kabobs uncovered 4 to 6 inches from medium heat 6 to 8 minutes, turning frequently and brushing several times with marinade, until shrimp are pink and firm. Discard any remaining marinade. Serve kabobs with orzo.

1 Serving:		% Daily Value:	
Calories	325	Vitamin A	10%
Calories from fat	20	Vitamin C	28%
Fat, g	2	Calcium	6%
Saturated, g	0	Iron	30%
Cholesterol, mg	160	**Diet Exchanges:**	
Sodium, mg	430	3 starch/bread	
Carbohydrate, g	56	1 lean meat	
Dietary Fiber, g	2	2 vegetable	
Protein, g	23		

Grilled Shrimp Kabobs

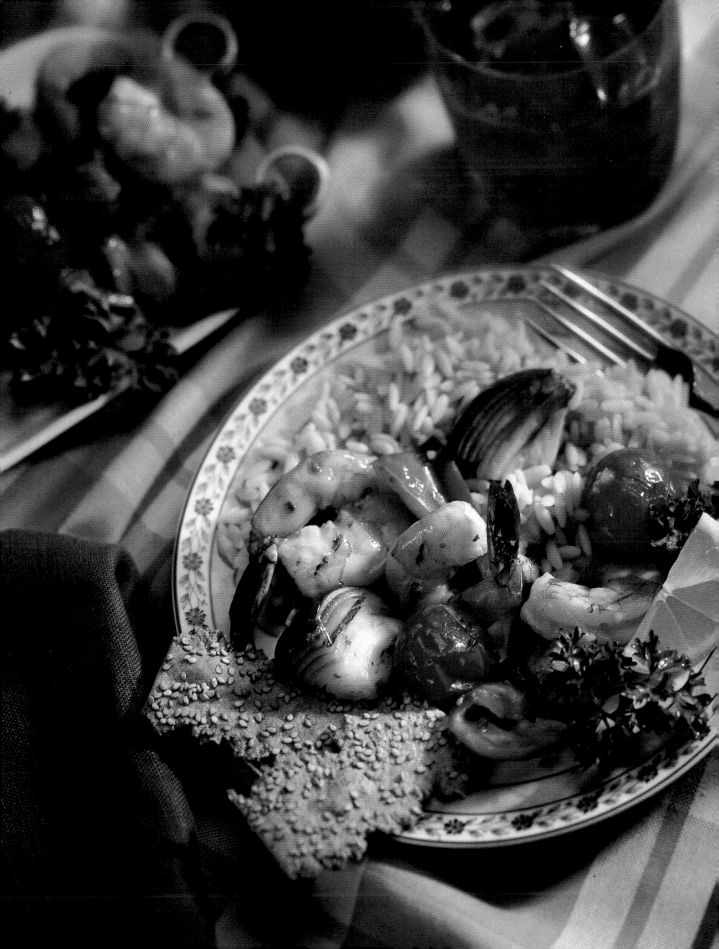

Ginger Shrimp and Vegetable Stir-Fry with Rice

PREP: 5 min; MARINATE: 45 min; COOK: 10 min

4 SERVINGS

Just a small amount of sesame oil brings the flavors of Asia to this easy stir-fry. It's worth buying a bottle for the extra flavor.

1/2 pound uncooked, peeled, deveined medium shrimp, thawed if frozen

1 tablespoon grated gingerroot

2 tablespoons reduced-sodium soy sauce

1 teaspoon sesame or vegetable oil

1/2 cup ready-to-serve fat-free reduced-sodium chicken broth

3 cups packaged fresh stir-fry vegetables

1 teaspoon cornstarch

4 cups hot cooked rice

Mix shrimp, gingerroot, soy sauce and oil in shallow nonmetal dish or heavy-duty resealable plastic bag. Cover dish or seal bag and refrigerate 45 minutes.

Heat 1/4 cup of the broth to boiling in wok or 10-inch nonstick skillet. Add stir-fry vegetables; stir-fry until liquid has evaporated. Add shrimp mixture; stir-fry 3 to 5 minutes or until shrimp are pink and firm. Mix cornstarch and remaining 1/4 cup broth; stir into shrimp mixture. Cook 1 minute or until sauce is thickened, stirring constantly. Serve over rice.

1 Serving:		% Daily Value:	
Calories	290	Vitamin A	14%
Calories from fat	25	Vitamin C	26%
Fat, g	3	Calcium	6%
Saturated, g	1	Iron	24%
Cholesterol, mg	80	**Diet Exchanges:**	
Sodium, mg	810	3 starch/bread	
Carbohydrate, g	53	1/2 lean meat	
Dietary Fiber, g	3	1 vegetable	
Protein, g	16		

Ginger Shrimp and Vegetable Stir-Fry with Rice

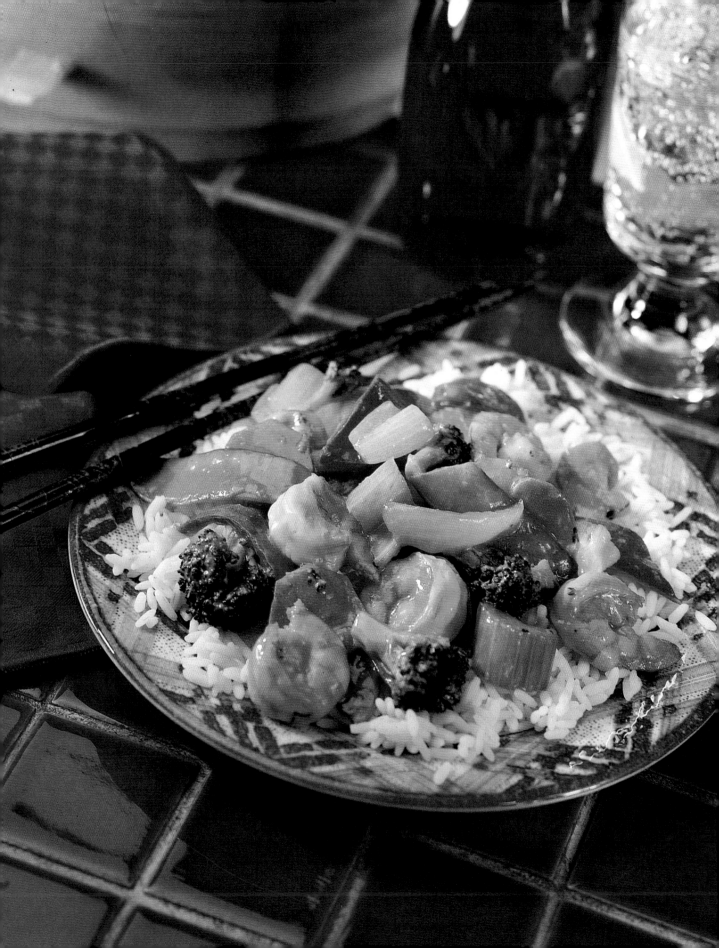

WATER: THE FORGOTTEN NUTRIENT

It may be hard to believe, but fully two-thirds of our bodies are comprised of water. A fact just as surprising is that, even with all that water, our bodies still need more water on a daily basis. How much water should we drink each day? Eight eight-ounce (one cup) glasses of water are recommended every day. Most of us don't drink enough. Other liquids can be counted toward the total amount, but don't count coffee or tea (regular or decaf) or alcoholic beverages; they have a dehydrating effect.

Drinking lots of water helps us in several ways. Not only does it keep the body hydrated and aid maintaining regularity, but it can also help maintain a healthier diet by filling you up and curbing hunger.

If you tend to forget about drinking water throughout the day, keep a pitcher or thermos of cold water by you and help yourself now and then during the day. If you want something warm and soothing, try sipping hot water with a fresh lemon wedge. Remember that you should drink water even when you are not thirsty; by the time you feel thirsty, it's a signal you're dehydrated. When you exercise, you need to increase your water consumption to make up for additional losses from sweat and heavier breathing.

Stir-Fried Garlic Shrimp

PREP: 10 min; COOK: 4 min

4 SERVINGS

2 teaspoons vegetable oil

1 pound uncooked, peeled, deveined medium shrimp, thawed if frozen

2 large cloves garlic, finely chopped

3 cups sliced mushrooms (8 ounces)

1 cup 1-inch pieces green onions

1/4 cup dry white wine or ready-to-serve fat-free reduced-sodium chicken broth

2 cups hot cooked rice

Heat oil in 10-inch nonstick skillet over medium-high heat. Add shrimp and garlic; stir-fry 1 minute. Add mushrooms, onions and wine; stir-fry about 2 minutes or until shrimp are pink and firm and vegetables are hot. Serve over rice.

1 Serving:		% Daily Value:	
Calories	225	Vitamin A	6%
Calories from fat	35	Vitamin C	6%
Fat, g	4	Calcium	6%
Saturated, g	1	Iron	26%
Cholesterol, mg	160	**Diet Exchanges:**	
Sodium, mg	190	1 1/2 starch/bread	
Carbohydrate, g	27	1 1/2 lean meat	
Dietary Fiber, g	1	1 vegetable	
Protein, g	21		

Lemon Shrimp-Vegetable Kabobs

PREP: 10 min; MARINATE: 30 min; BROIL: 8 min;
COOK: 2 min

4 SERVINGS

Serve the kabobs over rice with the boiled marinade as a tangy sauce.

1/2 pound uncooked, peeled, deveined medium shrimp, thawed if frozen

1/4 cup lemon juice

1 tablespoon balsamic or red wine vinegar

4 large cloves garlic, thinly sliced

1 medium zucchini, sliced (2 cups)

1 large red bell pepper, cut into eighths

2 teaspoons sesame or vegetable oil

Mix shrimp, lemon juice and vinegar in shallow nonmetal dish or heavy-duty resealable plastic bag. Cover dish or seal bag and refrigerate 30 minutes.

Remove shrimp from marinade; reserve marinade. Thread shrimp, garlic, zucchini and bell pepper alternately on each of eight 10- to 12-inch metal skewers. Brush with oil.

Set oven control to broil. Place kabobs on rack in broiler pan. Broil with tops 4 to 6 inches from heat about 8 minutes, turning once, until shrimp are pink and firm. Heat remaining marinade to boiling; boil and stir 1 minute. Serve marinade with kabobs.

1 Serving:		% Daily Value:	
Calories	65	Vitamin A	18%
Calories from fat	20	Vitamin C	46%
Fat, g	2	Calcium	2%
Saturated, g	0	Iron	8%
Cholesterol, mg	80	**Diet Exchanges:**	
Sodium, mg	95	1 lean meat	
Carbohydrate, g	4	1 vegetable	
Dietary Fiber, g	1		
Protein, g	9		

TRANS FATTY ACIDS: THE FACTS

What they are: Fatty acids form when vegetable oils are hydrogenated (hardened) but the location of the hydrogen molecules are in different spots than they naturally occur in solid or saturated fats. In short, their molecular structure has been altered. All margarines and hydrogenated vegetable oils contain trans fatty acids (butter does not contain trans fatty acids).

The claim: Several scientific studies have shown that high intakes of trans fatty acids can raise blood cholesterol levels and increase the risk of heart disease. Other research scientists disagree.

What you should know: What is known, after many years of research, is that a diet high in total fat increases the risk of certain diseases, such as heart disease. Until we have further scientific information, it is important to keep this issue in perspective. Therefore, the best dietary advice remains unchanged. As the U.S. Dietary Guidelines recommend: Increase intake of grains, fruits and vegetables, and reduce fat intake to 30 percent or calories or less and saturated fat to 10 percent of calories or less.

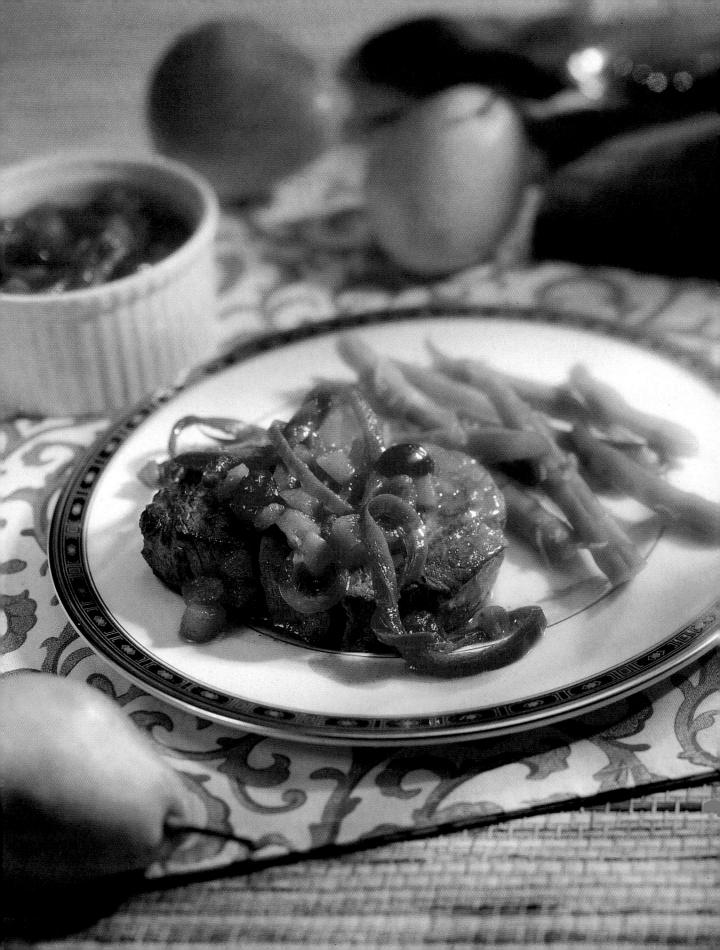

6

Great Beef, Pork and Lamb

Beef Medallions with Pear-Cranberry Chutney
(page 132)

Meat Loaf

PREP: 8 min; BAKE: 1 1/2 hr

8 SERVINGS

Lean ground turkey and old-fashioned oats help cut the fat but keep the moistness in this tasty version of a family favorite.

3/4 pound extra-lean ground beef

3/4 pound ground turkey breast

1/2 cup old-fashioned oats

1/2 cup tomato puree

2 tablespoons chopped fresh parsley

1/2 teaspoon Italian seasoning

1/2 teaspoon salt

1/4 teaspoon pepper

1 small onion, chopped (1/4 cup)

1 clove garlic, finely chopped

Heat oven to 350°. Mix all ingredients thoroughly. Press mixture evenly in ungreased loaf pan, 8 1/2 × 4 1/2 × 2 1/2 or 9 × 5 × 3 inches. Bake uncovered 1 1/4 to 1 1/2 hours or until no longer pink in center and juice is clear.

1 Serving:		% Daily Value:	
Calories	150	Vitamin A	2%
Calories from fat	55	Vitamin C	4%
Fat, g	6	Calcium	2%
Saturated, g	2	Iron	10%
Cholesterol, mg	50	**Diet Exchanges:**	
Sodium, mg	250	2 1/2 lean meat	
Carbohydrate, g	6	1 vegetable	
Dietary Fiber, g	1		
Protein, g	19		

Swiss Steak

PREP: 10 min; COOK: 1 3/4 hr

6 SERVINGS

1 1/2-pound beef boneless round, tip or chuck steak, about 3/4 inch thick

3 tablespoons all-purpose flour

1 teaspoon ground mustard (dry)

1/2 teaspoon salt

2 teaspoons vegetable oil

1 can (16 ounces) whole tomatoes, undrained

2 cloves garlic, finely chopped

1 cup water

1 large onion, sliced

1 large green bell pepper, sliced

Trim fat from beef. Mix flour, mustard and salt. Sprinkle one side of beef with half of the flour mixture; pound in. Turn beef and pound in remaining flour mixture. Cut beef into 6 serving pieces.

Heat oil in 10-inch nonstick skillet over medium heat. Cook beef in oil about 15 minutes, turning once, until brown. Add tomatoes and garlic, breaking up tomatoes. Heat to boiling; reduce heat to low. Cover and simmer about 1 1/4 hours or until beef is tender.

Add water, onion and bell pepper. Heat to boiling; reduce heat to medium. Cover and simmer 5 to 8 minutes or until vegetables are tender.

1 Serving:		% Daily Value:	
Calories	170	Vitamin A	6%
Calories from fat	45	Vitamin C	24%
Fat, g	5	Calcium	2%
Saturated, g	2	Iron	14%
Cholesterol, mg	55	**Diet Exchanges:**	
Sodium, mg	360	2 lean meat	
Carbohydrate, g	10	2 vegetable	
Dietary Fiber, g	1		
Protein, g	22		

Beef Tenderloin with Sweet Onions

PREP: 5 min; COOK: 20 min

4 SERVINGS

Balsamic vinegar and slow cooking give these onions melting sweetness—it's a guilt-free indulgence!

1/4 to 1/2 cup ready-to-serve fat-free reduced-sodium chicken broth

2 large onions, thinly sliced

4 cloves garlic, finely chopped

1/4 cup balsamic or cider vinegar

1/2 teaspoon salt

1/4 teaspoon freshly ground pepper

4 beef tenderloin steaks, about 1 inch thick (1 pound)

Heat 1/4 cup broth to boiling in 1-quart saucepan. Stir in onions and garlic; reduce heat to medium. Cover and cook about 15 minutes, stirring occasionally, until onions are very soft and brown, adding up to 1/4 cup more broth as needed to prevent onions from sticking. Stir in vinegar. Cook uncovered over medium-high heat about 2 minutes or until liquid has evaporated; remove from heat.

Meanwhile, spray 10-inch nonstick skillet with nonstick spray; heat over medium-high heat. Sprinkle salt and pepper on beef. Cook beef in skillet about 8 minutes for medium doneness, turning once.

1 Serving:		% Daily Value:	
Calories	180	Vitamin A	0%
Calories from fat	65	Vitamin C	4%
Fat, g	7	Calcium	2%
Saturated, g	3	Iron	12%
Cholesterol, mg	55	**Diet Exchanges:**	
Sodium, mg	370	3 lean meat	
Carbohydrate, g	8	1 vegetable	
Dietary Fiber, g	1		
Protein, g	22		

THE SKINNY ON CELLULITE

The fat that causes skin to take on a bumpy, orange-peel or cottage cheese–like appearance is called cellulite.

The makers of "cellulite-dissolving" creams, lotions and special massaging devices try to convince us that cellulite behaves differently than other types of body fat. But the truth is, it is all the same: Fat is fat. Fat cells are separated into compartments by strands of connective fiber directly under the skin. If the fat cells increase in size, they bulge out of these compartments giving the skin a bumpy appearance. Several factors influence this condition: the amount of fat in your body, the strength of the connective fibers and the thickness of the skin. Women tend to have tight fibers and thinner skin, so the fat between the fibers bulges more. Men, on the other hand, have flexible fibers and thicker skin, so their fat tends to be more evenly distributed. Some people are more prone to cellulite than others, and this may be in part genetic predisposition.

Contrary to popular belief, spot exercising will not reduce cellulite. No known magic creams, lotions or devices exist that will shrink cellulite. What will help is overall weight loss and getting regular aerobic exercise.

Beef Medallions with Pear-Cranberry Chutney

PREP: 8 min; COOK: 13 min

4 SERVINGS

Bright and tangy, this easy fruit chutney sets off the hearty beef. Serve leftover chutney cold on a turkey sandwich, or try it with chicken as well.

1 large red onion, thinly sliced

2 cloves garlic, finely chopped

2 tablespoons dry red wine or grape juice

2 firm ripe pears, peeled and diced

1/2 cup fresh or frozen cranberries

2 tablespoons packed brown sugar

1/2 teaspoon pumpkin pie spice

4 beef tenderloin steaks, about 1 inch thick (1 pound)

Spray 2-quart saucepan with nonstick cooking spray; heat over medium-high heat. Cook onion, garlic and wine in saucepan about 5 minutes, stirring frequently, until onion is tender but not brown. Stir in remaining ingredients except beef. Simmer uncovered, stirring frequently, until cranberries burst. Place chutney in small bowl; set aside.

Meanwhile, spray 10-inch nonstick skillet with nonstick cooking spray; heat over medium-high heat. Cook beef in skillet about 8 minutes, for medium doneness, turning once. Serve with chutney.

Pork Medallions: Trim fat from pork. Cut pork crosswise into 12 slices; flatten slightly. Follow directions above for Pear-Cranberry Chutney. Meanwhile, spray 10-inch nonstick skillet with nonstick cooking spray; heat over medium-high heat. Cook pork in skillet about 8 to 10 minutes, turning once, or until pork is slightly pink in center. Serve with chutney.

1 Serving:		% Daily Value:	
Calories	225	Vitamin A	0%
Calories from fat	65	Vitamin C	4%
Fat, g	7	Calcium	2%
Saturated, g	3	Iron	12%
Cholesterol, mg	55	**Diet Exchanges:**	
Sodium, mg	55	2 1/2 lean meat	
Carbohydrate, g	23	1 1/2 fruit	
Dietary Fiber, g	3		
Protein, g	21		

Skewered Steak Dinner

PREP: 12 min; MARINATE: 1 hr; GRILL: 20 min

6 SERVINGS

1 1/2 pounds beef boneless sirloin, cut into 1-inch cubes

1/2 cup fat-free Italian dressing

1 medium onion, cut into 6 wedges

1 medium green bell pepper, cut into 1 1/2 × 1-inch chunks

6 cherry tomatoes

Place beef and dressing in heavy-duty resealable plastic bag. Seal bag and refrigerate at least 1 hour but no longer than 24 hours.

Heat coals or gas grill for direct heat. Remove beef from marinade; reserve marinade. Thread beef, onion and bell pepper alternately on each of six 15-inch metal skewers, leaving about 1/4 inch between each piece. Place 1 cherry tomato on end of each skewer. Brush kabobs generously with marinade.

Cover and grill kabobs 4 to 6 inches from medium heat 15 to 20 minutes for medium beef doneness, turning kabobs frequently and brushing with marinade. Discard any remaining marinade.

1 Serving:		% Daily Value:	
Calories	125	Vitamin A	2%
Calories from fat	25	Vitamin C	12%
Fat, g	3	Calcium	0%
Saturated, g	2	Iron	10%
Cholesterol, mg	55	**Diet Exchanges:**	
Sodium, mg	160	2 lean meat	
Carbohydrate, g	5	1 vegetable	
Dietary Fiber, g	1		
Protein, g	20		

Mexican Flank Steak

PREP: 10 min; MARINATE: 8 hr; BROIL: 10 min; COOK: 2 min

6 SERVINGS

1 pound lean beef flank steak

1/3 cup lime juice

1 teaspoon vegetable oil

1/2 teaspoon salt

1 small onion, chopped (1/4 cup)

2 cloves garlic, finely chopped

1 can (4 ounces) chopped green chilies, undrained

Trim fat from beef. Cut both sides of beef into diamond pattern 1/8 inch deep. Place in nonmetal dish or heavy-duty resealable plastic bag. Mix remaining ingredients; pour over beef, turning beef to coat both sides with marinade. Cover and refrigerate at least 8 hours but no longer than 24 hours, turning occasionally.

Set oven control to broil. Drain and scrape marinade off of beef; reserve marinade. Broil beef with top 2 to 3 inches from heat 10 minutes for medium doneness, turning once. Cut beef diagonally across grain into thin slices. Heat marinade to boiling; boil and stir 1 minute. Serve marinade with beef.

1 Serving:		% Daily Value:	
Calories	125	Vitamin A	0%
Calories from fat	55	Vitamin C	14%
Fat, g	6	Calcium	0%
Saturated, g	2	Iron	8%
Cholesterol, mg	40	**Diet Exchanges:**	
Sodium, mg	460	2 lean meat	
Carbohydrate, g	3	1 vegetable	
Dietary Fiber, g	0		
Protein, g	15		

Mexican Steak Stir-Fry

<small>PREP: 12 min; COOK: 10 min</small>

4 SERVINGS

Serve this over cooked rice or orzo pasta.

**3/4 pound beef boneless sirloin, cut into
  1 × 1/2-inch pieces**

1 medium onion, chopped (1/2 cup)

1 small green bell pepper, chopped (1/2 cup)

1 cup frozen whole kernel corn

1/2 cup salsa

1 medium zucchini, sliced (2 cups)

**1 can (15 to 16 ounces) pinto beans, rinsed
  and drained**

**1 can (14 1/2 ounces) no-salt-added whole
  tomatoes, undrained**

Spray 12-inch nonstick skillet with nonstick cooking spray; heat over medium-high heat. Cook beef, onion and bell pepper in skillet 4 to 5 minutes, stirring frequently, until beef is no longer pink.

Stir in remaining ingredients, breaking up tomatoes. Cook about 5 minutes, stirring occasionally, until zucchini is tender and mixture is hot.

1 Serving:		% Daily Value:	
Calories	270	Vitamin A	12%
Calories from fat	35	Vitamin C	34%
Fat, g	4	Calcium	10%
Saturated, g	1	Iron	28%
Cholesterol, mg	45	**Diet Exchanges:**	
Sodium, mg	360	2 starch/bread	
Carbohydrate, g	42	1 1/2 lean meat	
Dietary Fiber, g	12	2 vegetable	
Protein, g	28		

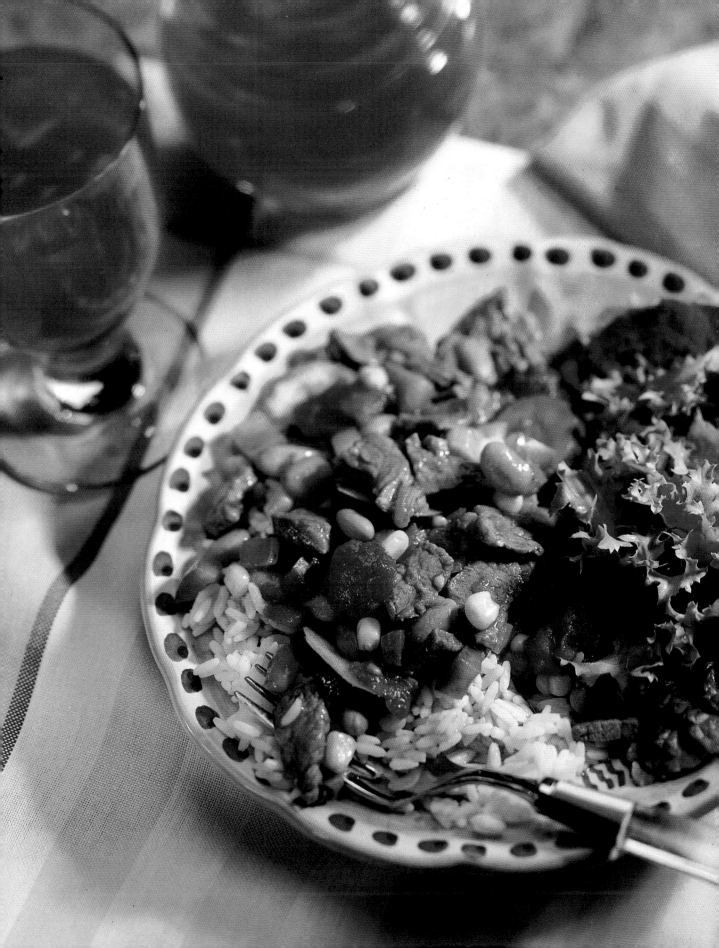

Garlicky Meatballs Over Rice

PREP: 10 min; COOK: 30 min

4 SERVINGS

If you love garlic and chilies, these are the meatballs for you!

3/4 pound extra-lean ground beef

1 slice whole wheat bread, crumbled

1/4 cup salsa

4 cloves garlic, finely chopped

2 cans (8 ounces each) tomato sauce

3 cups hot cooked rice

Mix all ingredients except tomato sauce and rice. Shape into sixteen 1 1/2-inch meatballs.

Spray 10-inch nonstick skillet with nonstick cooking spray; heat over medium-high heat. Place meatballs in skillet; spray meatballs with nonstick cooking spray. Cook until meatballs are brown on all sides.

Stir in tomato sauce. Heat to boiling; reduce heat to low. Cover and simmer about 20 minutes, stirring occasionally until meatballs are are no longer pink in center. Serve over rice:

1 Serving:		% Daily Value:	
Calories	355	Vitamin A	12%
Calories from fat	90	Vitamin C	16%
Fat, g	10	Calcium	4%
Saturated, g	4	Iron	24%
Cholesterol, mg	50	**Diet Exchanges:**	
Sodium, mg	810	3 starch/bread	
Carbohydrate, g	47	2 lean meat	
Dietary Fiber, g	3		
Protein, g	22		

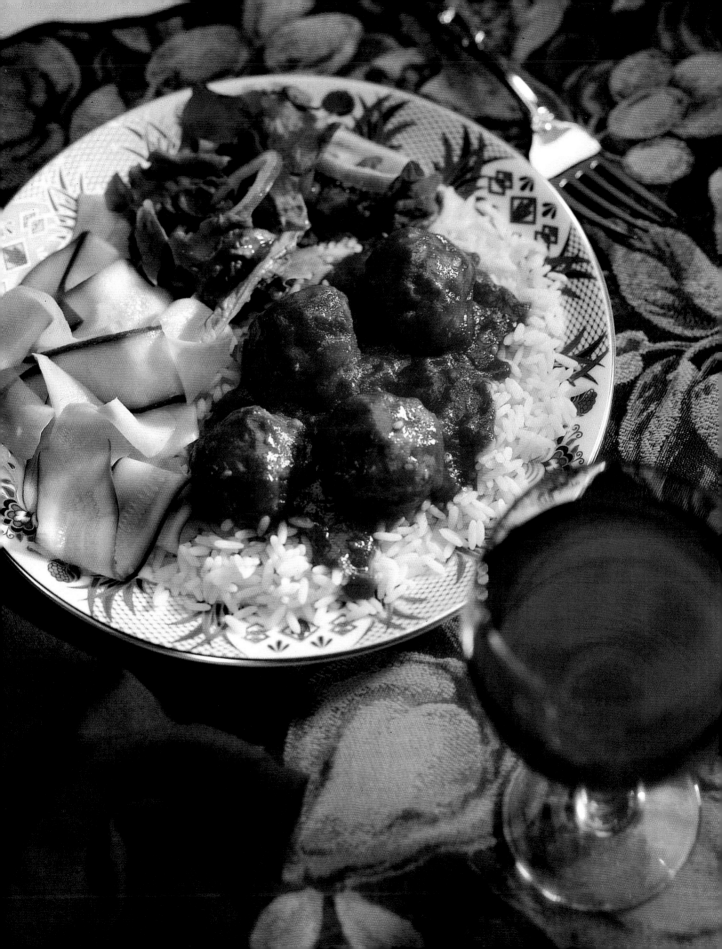

Solutions for Problem Eating

Problem	Solution
Eating too fast	• Try to allow 25 to 30 minutes for each meal. It takes our stomach 20 minutes to get the signal from our brain that it's full. • Take smaller bites and chew thoroughly and slowly.
Nibbling and snacking	• Don't skip meals; you will get too hungry and may overeat or eat high-calorie/high-fat foods. Eat 3 meals daily and 1 or 2 low-calorie/low-fat snacks. • Talk to yourself before eating something you really feel bad about and ask why you want to eat it. Convince yourself it's not worth feeling bad about. • Wait at least 10 minutes before eating anything unplanned.
Tempting food: Each of us has "trouble" foods that we just can't say no to.	The best way not to eat these is to eliminate them from your home completely.
That time of day: Problem times of the day, when we really seem to get the munchies or cravings, affect all of us.	When the clock strikes, strike back by getting moving, drink a glass of water or hot tea or help yourself to a healthful snack that you've preplanned.

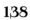

Problem	Solution
That time of month: Women often have preperiod cravings, and most women don't crave celery sticks—but chocolate or sweets! Often, ignoring an intense craving leads to overeating, so the key is to be in control and allow yourself to indulge in your craving in a smarter, small-scale way. So instead of eating a candy bar, cookies, cake or pie, try the suggestions below.	If you stick to your eating plan otherwise, these little treats won't get you off track. • 2 or 3 chocolate kisses • 2 or 3 hard candies • 1 or 2 pieces licorice • 1/2 cup frozen low-fat or fat-free yogurt or ice cream • 6 ounces chocolate yogurt • 1 small container ready-to-eat fat-free chocolate pudding
I'm eating because I'm • depressed • stressed out • bored • anxious • frustrated • tired • excited • in crisis • alone	Emotion acts as a powerful trigger to eat, but there are ways to counteract that effect. • Become aware of and record your feelings—look for patterns. • Talk to someone about your feelings. • Engage in an activity to take your mind off food. Take a walk, talk to a friend, write a letter, water the plants. More often than not, these diversions will make the original urge much, much weaker.
Eating events such as the holidays and parties.	• Don't go to the event hungry. Eat a piece of fruit, small salad or drink a large glass or water before arriving. • Have a plan to limit what types of food you eat and how much and stick to it. Don't go back for seconds. • Concentrate on low-fat food options such as fresh fruit and vegetables. • Have fun talking to people!

Chili-Stuffed Peppers

PREP: 8 min; COOK: 25 min; BAKE: 45 min

4 SERVINGS

4 large red or green bell peppers

1/2 pound extra-lean ground beef

1 medium onion, finely chopped (1/2 cup)

1 can (15 to 16 ounces) kidney beans, rinsed and drained

1 can (15 ounces) tomato puree

1 can (4 ounces) chopped green chilies, undrained

2 teaspoons chili powder

1/2 teaspoon ground cumin

Heat oven to 350°. Cut bell peppers lengthwise in half. Remove stems and seeds. Place peppers, cut sides up, in ungreased rectangular baking dish, 13 × 9 × 2 inches.

Cook beef and onion in 10-inch nonstick skillet over medium heat, stirring occasionally, until beef is brown; drain. Stir in remaining ingredients. Heat to boiling; reduce heat to low. Cover and simmer 10 minutes, stirring frequently.

Divide beef mixture evenly among peppers. Cover and bake 40 to 45 minutes or until peppers are tender.

1 Serving:		% Daily Value:	
Calories	250	Vitamin A	78%
Calories from fat	65	Vitamin C	100%
Fat, g	7	Calcium	6%
Saturated, g	3	Iron	28%
Cholesterol, mg	35	**Diet Exchanges:**	
Sodium, mg	1120	2 starch/bread	
Carbohydrate, g	36	1 lean meat	
Dietary Fiber, g	9	1 vegetable	
Protein, g	20		

Pork with Basil

PREP: 10 min; COOK: 12 min

4 SERVINGS

3/4 pound lean pork tenderloin

1 teaspoon vegetable oil

1/4 cup chopped fresh or 1 teaspoon dried basil leaves

1/4 cup ready-to-serve fat-free reduced-sodium chicken broth

1/8 teaspoon ground red pepper (cayenne)

4 cloves garlic, finely chopped

Trim fat from pork. Cut pork crosswise into 8 pieces. Flatten each piece to 1/4-inch thickness between waxed paper or plastic wrap.

Heat oil in 10-inch nonstick skillet over medium-high heat. Cook pork in oil about 4 minutes, turning once, until brown. Stir in remaining ingredients. Heat to boiling; reduce heat to low. Cover and simmer about 5 minutes or until pork is slightly pink in center.

1 Serving:		% Daily Value:	
Calories	115	Vitamin A	0%
Calories from fat	35	Vitamin C	0%
Fat, g	4	Calcium	0%
Saturated, g	1	Iron	6%
Cholesterol, mg	55	**Diet Exchanges:**	
Sodium, mg	65	2 lean meat	
Carbohydrate, g	1		
Dietary Fiber, g	0		
Protein, g	19		

SURVIVING THE HOLIDAYS

Traditional holiday meals can pack quite a caloric and fat-laden punch! However, you can still eat your favorite foods with some simple recipe modifications and attention to portion control. We've shown you below how to navigate a Thanksgiving meal, but the same principles would apply to any holiday meal or special-occasion meal:

Appetizers: Stick to fresh vegetables, fruit, shrimp, crab and pretzels. Avoid the dips, spreads (unless made with fat-free or low-fat products), creamy and cheesy mixtures and fried foods. Try our Tangy Yogurt Dip (page 32) with fresh vegetables and Gorgonzola and Caramelized Onion Appetizer (page 42).

Roast Turkey: Eat white meat without the skin. If you're having a very small group of people, try Maple-Roasted Chicken with Wild Rice Stuffing (page 98) instead of turkey.

Stuffing: Cook the vegetables in broth instead of butter or margarine. Skip the sausage and bake the stuffing in a casserole rather than inside the bird; this will prevent extra fat from absorbing into the stuffing.

Mashed Potatoes: Mash potatoes with skim milk and no fat. Flavored mashed potatoes add pizzazz without fat. Try adding garlic cloves to the cooking water or stir chopped fresh chives or horseradish into mashed potatoes. For buttery flavor, try butter-flavored sprinkles or packets that are mixed with water and used like melted butter.

Gravy: Use a fat strainer to separate the juices from the fat. For richer gravy, stir in evaporated skim milk before thickening.

Green Bean Casserole: Use a reduced-fat cream soup and skim milk. Sprinkle top with only 2 tablespoons fried onions—if the onions are crushed after measuring they will stretch further. Another option is to top the beans with crushed reduced-fat potato chips. Or, for a change of pace, prepare Green Beans with Pimiento Sauce (page 205).

Sweet Potato Casserole: Top sweet potatoes with 2 tablespoons brown sugar or honey and 1/2 cup miniature marshmallows; skip the butter. Whole baked sweet potatoes are delicious, too, especially Sweet Potatoes with Onion Topping (page 204).

Pumpkin Pie: Use evaporated skim milk and cholesterol-free, fat-free egg product for the filling and skip the crust. A crust isn't necessary for successful results, but because it may get done more quickly, check for doneness five to ten minutes earlier than indicated in the recipe. Top with fat-free or light whipped topping instead of whipped cream. Cut the pie into eight or ten pieces. Pumpkin Molasses Cheesecakes (page 228) are so easy to make and each person gets his or her own little dessert.

Grilled Southwestern Pork Chops

PREP: 5 min; CHILL: 1 hr; GRILL: 12 min

8 SERVINGS

8 pork loin or rib chops, about 1/2 inch thick (2 pounds)

1 tablespoon chili powder

1 teaspoon ground cumin

1/4 teaspoon ground red pepper (cayenne)

1/4 teaspoon salt

1 large clove garlic, finely chopped

Trim fat from pork. Mix remaining ingredients. Rub chili powder mixture evenly on both sides of pork. Cover and refrigerate 1 hour to blend flavors.

Heat coals or gas grill for direct heat. Cover and grill pork 4 to 6 inches from medium heat 10 to 12 minutes, turning frequently, until slightly pink when cut near bone.

1 Serving:		% Daily Value:	
Calories	170	Vitamin A	4%
Calories from fat	70	Vitamin C	0%
Fat, g	8	Calcium	0%
Saturated, g	3	Iron	6%
Cholesterol, mg	65	**Diet Exchanges:**	
Sodium, mg	120	3 lean meat	
Carbohydrate, g	1		
Dietary Fiber, g	0		
Protein, g	23		

Zesty Pork Tenderloin

PREP: 5 min; MARINATE: 1 hr; ROAST: 29 min

6 SERVINGS

1/4 cup ketchup

1 tablespoon sugar

1 tablespoon dry white wine or water

1 tablespoon hoisin sauce

1 clove garlic, finely chopped

2 pork tenderloins (about 3/4 pound each)

Mix all ingredients except pork in heavy-duty resealable plastic bag. Add pork, turning to coat with marinade. Seal bag and refrigerate at least 1 hour but no longer than 24 hours.

Heat oven to 425°. Place pork with marinade on rack in shallow roasting pan. Insert meat thermometer horizontally so tip is in thickest part of pork. Roast uncovered 27 to 29 minutes or until thermometer reads 160° (medium doneness).

1 Serving:		% Daily Value:	
Calories	155	Vitamin A	2%
Calories from fat	35	Vitamin C	2%
Fat, g	4	Calcium	0%
Saturated, g	2	Iron	8%
Cholesterol, mg	65	**Diet Exchanges:**	
Sodium, mg	170	2 1/2 lean meat	
Carbohydrate, g	6	1/2 fruit	
Dietary Fiber, g	0		
Protein, g	24		

Zesty Pork Tenderloin

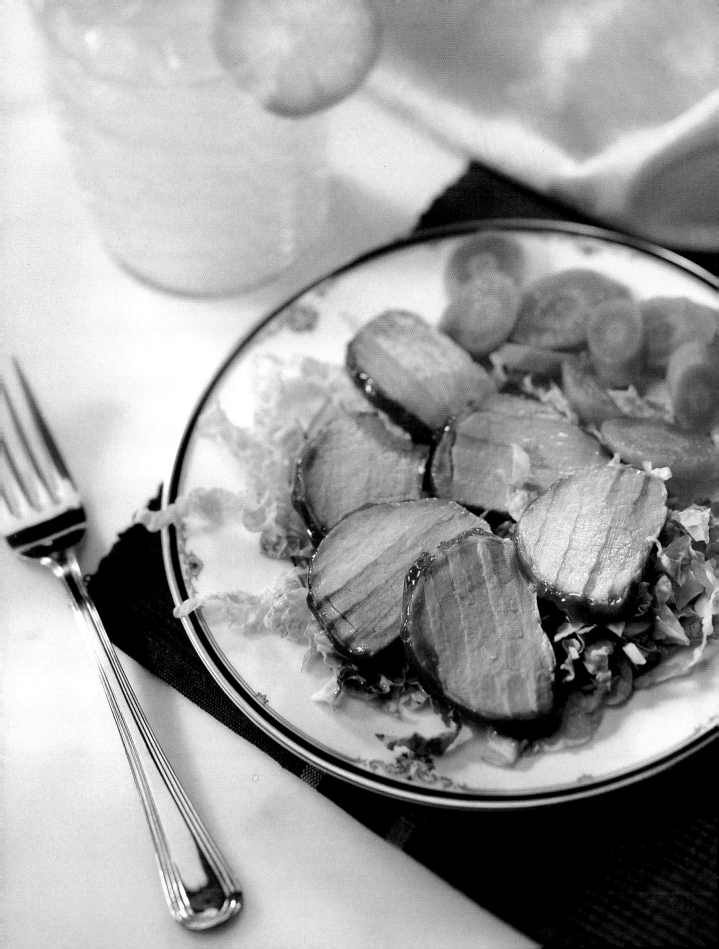

Southwestern Pork and Potato Stew

PREP: 15 min; COOK: 40 min

4 SERVINGS

The flavors of the Southwest inspired this savory stew. It's very good served with rice.

1 pound lean pork boneless shoulder

2 1/4 cups ready-to-serve fat-free reduced-sodium chicken broth

1 medium onion, chopped (1/2 cup)

3 cloves garlic, finely chopped

3 cups frozen green beans, potatoes and red peppers (from 16-ounce package)

1 teaspoon dried thyme leaves

1/2 teaspoon ground cumin

2 tablespoons chopped fresh or canned jalapeño chilies

Trim fat from pork. Cut pork into 1-inch cubes. Spray Dutch oven with nonstick cooking spray; heat over medium-high heat. Cook pork in Dutch oven, stirring occasionally, until brown.

Stir in 1/2 cup of the broth, the onion and garlic. Cook 5 minutes. Stir in vegetable mixture, remaining 1 3/4 cups broth, the thyme, cumin and chilies. Heat to boiling; reduce heat to low. Cover and simmer about 25 minutes or until pork is slightly pink in center.

1 Serving:		% Daily Value:	
Calories	215	Vitamin A	2%
Calories from fat	80	Vitamin C	8%
Fat, g	9	Calcium	4%
Saturated, g	4	Iron	10%
Cholesterol, mg	50	**Diet Exchanges:**	
Sodium, mg	330	1 starch/bread	
Carbohydrate, g	17	2 1/2 lean meat	
Dietary Fiber, g	3		
Protein, g	19		

Pineapple Pork Chops

PREP: 5 min; MARINATE: 1 hr; COOK: 31 min

4 SERVINGS

Marinate the chops overnight or during the day, then you can make a quick dinner.

4 lean pork loin or rib chops, about 1/2 inch thick (about 1 pound)

3 cloves garlic, finely chopped

1 can (8 ounces) crushed pineapple in juice, undrained

1 tablespoon honey mustard

1/4 teaspoon salt

Trim fat from pork. Mix garlic, pineapple and mustard in heavy-duty resealable plastic bag. Add pork, turning to coat with marinade. Seal bag and refrigerate at least 1 hour but no longer than 24 hours.

Remove pork from marinade; reserve marinade. Spray 10-inch nonstick skillet with nonstick cooking spray; heat over medium-high heat. Cook pork in skillet about 6 minutes, turning once, until brown. Sprinkle with salt and add marinade; reduce heat to low. Cover and simmer about 10 to 12 minutes or until pork is slightly pink when cut near bone.

1 Serving:		% Daily Value:	
Calories	205	Vitamin A	0%
Calories from fat	70	Vitamin C	4%
Fat, g	8	Calcium	2%
Saturated, g	3	Iron	6%
Cholesterol, mg	65	**Diet Exchanges:**	
Sodium, mg	230	3 lean meat	
Carbohydrate, g	10	1/2 fruit	
Dietary Fiber, g	0		
Protein, g	23		

Pineapple Pork Chops

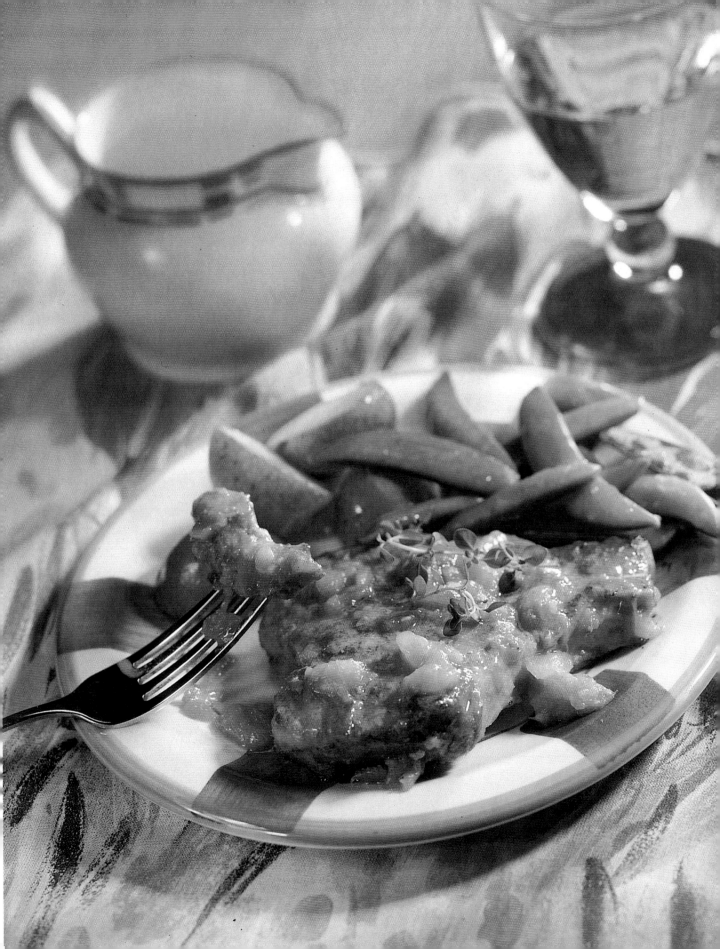

Pork, Onion and Pepper Fajitas

PREP: 10 min; MARINATE: 8 hr; COOK: 11 min

4 SERVINGS

Garnish these fast fajitas with chopped tomato, cilantro, reduced-fat sour cream or yogurt, and salsa.

1/2 pound pork tenderloin

1/4 cup lime juice

1 1/2 teaspoons ground cumin

3/4 teaspoon salt

4 cloves garlic, finely chopped

1 large onion, thinly sliced

3 medium bell peppers, thinly sliced

4 fat-free flour tortillas (6 to 8 inches in diameter)

Trim fat from pork; cut into 2 × 1/2-inch strips. Mix lime juice, cumin, salt, garlic and pork in heavy-duty resealable plastic bag. Seal bag and refrigerate at least 8 hours but no longer than 24 hours.

Remove pork from marinade; reserve marinade. Spray 10-inch skillet with nonstick cooking spray; heat over medium-high heat. Cook pork in skillet 3 minutes, stirring once. Stir in onion, bell peppers and marinade. Cook 5 to 8 minutes, stirring occasionally, until onion and peppers are crisp-tender.

Place one-fourth of the pork mixture in center of each tortilla. Fold one end of tortilla up about 1 inch over pork mixture; fold right and left sides over folded end, overlapping. Fold remaining end down.

1 Serving:		% Daily Value:	
Calories	220	Vitamin A	4%
Calories from fat	25	Vitamin C	46%
Fat, g	3	Calcium	8%
Saturated, g	1	Iron	16%
Cholesterol, mg	35	**Diet Exchanges:**	
Sodium, mg	670	2 starch/bread	
Carbohydrate, g	33	1 lean meat	
Dietary Fiber, g	3	1 vegetable	
Protein, g	18		

Ham- and Swiss-Topped Potatoes

PREP: 5 min; BAKE: 1 hr; COOK: 7 min

6 SERVINGS

Want to shorten the cooking time on the potatoes? Zap them in the microwave on High for 10 to 13 minutes.

3 medium baking potatoes

2 tablespoons cornstarch

2 cups skim milk

1 tablespoon Dijon mustard

1/4 teaspoon pepper

1/2 cup shredded reduced-fat Swiss cheese (2 ounces)

1/2 pound deli-style sliced fat-free ham, cut into 1/2-inch strips (2 cups)

1 package (10 ounces) frozen asparagus cuts, thawed and drained

Heat oven to 375°. Prick potatoes with fork. Bake about 1 hour or until tender.

Mix cornstarch and milk in 2-quart nonstick saucepan. Cook over medium heat, stirring constantly, until mixture thickens and boils. Stir in mustard, pepper and cheese until cheese is melted. Stir in ham and asparagus; heat through. Cut potatoes lengthwise in half. Serve sauce over potato halves.

1 Serving:		% Daily Value:	
Calories	170	Vitamin A	8%
Calories from fat	35	Vitamin C	20%
Fat, g	4	Calcium	22%
Saturated, g	2	Iron	6%
Cholesterol, mg	25	**Diet Exchanges:**	
Sodium, mg	550	1 starch/bread	
Carbohydrate, g	19	1 1/2 lean meat	
Dietary Fiber, g	1	1 vegetable	
Protein, g	16		

Lamb with Yogurt-Mint Sauce

PREP: 5 min; BROIL: 14 min

4 SERVINGS

2/3 cup plain fat-free yogurt

1/4 cup firmly packed fresh mint leaves

2 tablespoons sugar

4 lamb loin chops, about 1 inch thick (1 pound)

Place yogurt, mint and sugar in blender or food processor. Cover and blend on medium speed, stopping blender occasionally to scrape sides, until leaves are finely chopped.

Set oven control to broil. Spray broiler pan rack with nonstick cooking spray. Trim fat from lamb. Place lamb on rack in broiler pan. Broil with tops 2 to 3 inches from heat 12 to 14 minutes for medium (160°), turning after 6 minutes. Serve with sauce.

1 Serving:		% Daily Value:	
Calories	170	Vitamin A	0%
Calories from fat	55	Vitamin C	0%
Fat, g	6	Calcium	8%
Saturated, g	2	Iron	8%
Cholesterol, mg	60	**Diet Exchanges:**	
Sodium, mg	75	3 lean meat	
Carbohydrate, g	9	1/2 fruit	
Dietary Fiber, g	0		
Protein, g	20		

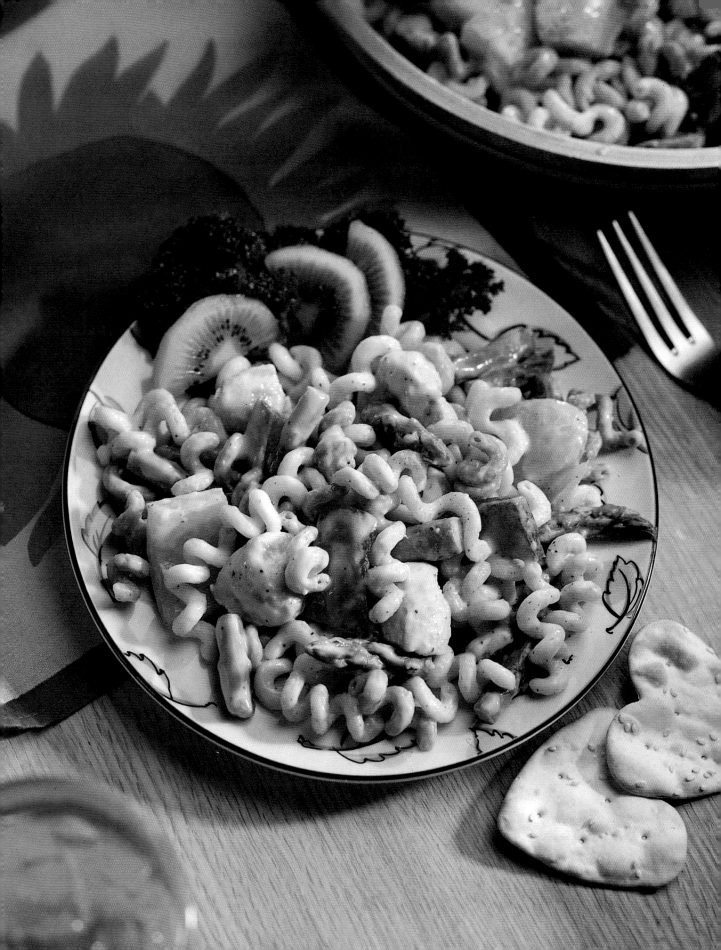

7

Pasta and Pizza with Pizzazz

Chicken-Fusilli-Vegetable Toss
(page 152)

Pizza Casserole

PREP: 8 min; COOK: 12 min; BAKE: 30 min;
STAND: 5 min

6 SERVINGS

**4 cups uncooked wagon wheel pasta
(8 ounces)**

1/2 pound bulk turkey Italian sausage

1/4 cup sliced ripe olives

**1 can (4 ounces) mushroom stems and
pieces, drained**

**1 jar (26 to 28 ounces) fat-free spaghetti
sauce**

**1 cup shredded reduced-fat mozzarella
cheese (4 ounces)**

Heat oven to 350°. Cook and drain pasta as directed
on package. Cook sausage in 10-inch skillet over
medium-high heat, stirring frequently, until no
longer pink; drain. Mix pasta, sausage and remaining ingredients except cheese in ungreased
2 1/2-quart casserole.

Cover and bake about 30 minutes or until hot.
Sprinkle with cheese. Cover and let stand about
5 minutes or until cheese is melted.

1 Serving:		% Daily Value:	
Calories	315	Vitamin A	4%
Calories from fat	80	Vitamin C	0%
Fat, g	9	Calcium	16%
Saturated, g	4	Iron	12%
Cholesterol, mg	40	**Diet Exchanges:**	
Sodium, mg	950	2 starch/bread	
Carbohydrate, g	42	2 lean meat	
Dietary Fiber, g	4	2 vegetable	
Protein, g	20		

Fiery Fettuccine

PREP: 8 min; COOK: 13 min

4 SERVINGS

8 ounces uncooked fettuccine

**2 1/2 cups evaporated skimmed milk or
fat-free half-and-half**

2 tablespoons all-purpose flour

1 tablespoon Creole or Cajun seasoning

**1 jar (7 1/4 ounces) roasted red bell peppers,
drained**

**1/4 pound fat-free smoked sausage ring, cut
into 1/2-inch pieces (from 16-ounce
ring)**

2 medium green onions, sliced (1/4 cup)

Cook and drain fettuccine as directed on package.
While fettuccine is cooking, place milk, flour,
Creole seasoning and bell peppers in blender or
food processor. Cover and blend on high speed
until smooth.

Pour pepper mixture into 12-inch nonstick skillet.
Cook over medium heat, stirring occasionally, until
thickened. Stir in sausage; heat through but do
not boil. Serve sausage mixture over fettuccine.
Sprinkle with onions.

1 Serving:		% Daily Value:	
Calories	380	Vitamin A	36%
Calories from fat	25	Vitamin C	54%
Fat, g	3	Calcium	50%
Saturated, g	1	Iron	18%
Cholesterol, mg	65	**Diet Exchanges:**	
Sodium, mg	650	4 starch/bread	
Carbohydrate, g	66	1/2 skim milk	
Dietary Fiber, g	2		
Protein, g	24		

Chicken-Basil Noodles

PREP: 10 min; COOK: 10 min

4 SERVINGS

2 teaspoons olive or vegetable oil

1 medium onion, finely chopped (1/2 cup)

1 clove garlic, finely chopped

3 medium tomatoes, seeded and chopped (2 1/4 cups)

2 cups cubed cooked chicken or turkey breast

1/4 cup chopped fresh basil leaves

1/2 teaspoon salt

2 cups uncooked cholesterol-free noodles (4 ounces)

Heat oil in 10-inch nonstick skillet over medium-high heat. Cook onion and garlic in oil, stirring occasionally, until onion is tender. Stir in remaining ingredients except noodles; reduce heat to medium.

Cover and cook about 5 minutes, stirring frequently, until mixture is hot and tomatoes are soft. Meanwhile, cook and drain noodles as directed on package. Serve chicken mixture over noodles.

1 Serving:		% Daily Value:	
Calories	240	Vitamin A	8%
Calories from fat	45	Vitamin C	20%
Fat, g	5	Calcium	4%
Saturated, g	1	Iron	14%
Cholesterol, mg	50	**Diet Exchanges:**	
Sodium, mg	350	1 starch/bread	
Carbohydrate, g	26	2 lean meat	
Dietary Fiber, g	2	2 vegetable	
Protein, g	25		

DOES PASTA MAKE YOU FAT?

First we hear how good pasta is for you; then, headlines and television news stories tell us that pasta makes you fat. The claim is that pasta boosts insulin levels and causes weight gain. So what is the truth about pasta? The truth is, there's no need to avoid eating pasta.

After eating, blood sugar (glucose) levels rise in our bodies, causing insulin, a component necessary to break down carbohydrates, to be released into the bloodstream. Insulin helps body cells take in and store glucose as energy. In insulin-resistant people, the cells are not as sensitive to insulin so the body continues to make more, which eventually can result in diabetes. It isn't the insulin resistance that causes weight gain, but rather, obesity causes insulin resistance, which may increase risk for other diseases, such as high blood pressure, heart disease and diabetes.

Pasta is not a big problem for people who are insulin resistant, since it raises blood sugar only moderately. Experts in nutrition still recommend a diet low in fat and rich in carbohydrates. Your best bet is to eat less fat, count calories (any extra calories are stored as fat), choose foods high in fiber such as whole grains, legumes and vegetables, and stay active as exercise tones muscles and balances calorie intake.

Chicken-Fusilli-Vegetable Toss

PREP: 10 min; COOK: 13 min

6 SERVINGS

To save time, try using one 10-ounce package frozen asparagus cuts and 2 cups frozen bell pepper chunks instead of cutting up fresh vegetables.

3 cups uncooked fusilli pasta (9 ounces)

3/4 pound skinless boneless chicken breast halves, cut into 1-inch pieces

1 medium red bell pepper, cut into 1-inch pieces

1 medium yellow bell pepper, cut into 1-inch pieces

1/2 pound asparagus, cut into 1-inch pieces

1 tablespoon water

1/2 teaspoon pepper

1 container (10 ounces) refrigerated reduced-fat Alfredo sauce

Cook and drain pasta as directed on package. While pasta is cooking, spray 12-inch skillet with nonstick cooking spray; heat over medium-high heat. Cook chicken in skillet 3 to 4 minutes, stirring frequently, until brown.

Stir in bell peppers, asparagus, water and pepper; reduce heat to low. Cover and simmer 3 to 4 minutes, stirring occasionally, until chicken is no longer pink in center and vegetables are crisp-tender. Toss pasta, chicken mixture and Alfredo sauce; heat through.

1 Serving:		% Daily Value:	
Calories	290	Vitamin A	8%
Calories from fat	70	Vitamin C	42%
Fat, g	8	Calcium	2%
Saturated, g	4	Iron	12%
Cholesterol, mg	50	**Diet Exchanges:**	
Sodium, mg	260	2 starch/bread	
Carbohydrate, g	36	2 lean meat	
Dietary Fiber, g	2	1 vegetable	
Protein, g	21		

Oriental Ginger Chicken

PREP: 8 min; COOK: 10 min

6 SERVINGS

Fresh gingerroot adds delightful flavor and aroma to this dish. For fresh ginger anytime, store it in the freezer and grate while frozen.

3 cups uncooked rotini pasta (9 ounces)

1 pound skinless boneless chicken breast halves, cut into 1/2-inch strips

1 package (16 ounces) frozen broccoli, water chestnuts and red peppers

3/4 cup sweet-and-sour sauce

1 tablespoon finely chopped fresh ginger-root or 1/2 teaspoon ground ginger

Cook and drain pasta as directed on package. While pasta is cooking, spray 12-inch skillet with nonstick cooking spray; heat over medium-high heat. Cook chicken in skillet 2 to 3 minutes, stirring frequently, until brown. Stir in remaining ingredients; reduce heat to low. Cover and simmer 3 to 4 minutes or until chicken is no longer pink in center and vegetables are crisp-tender. Toss with pasta.

1 Serving:		% Daily Value:	
Calories	290	Vitamin A	8%
Calories from fat	35	Vitamin C	20%
Fat, g	4	Calcium	4%
Saturated, g	1	Iron	16%
Cholesterol, mg	40	**Diet Exchanges:**	
Sodium, mg	420	2 starch/bread	
Carbohydrate, g	44	1 1/2 lean meat	
Dietary Fiber, g	3	1 fruit	
Protein, g	23		

Vegetable-Sausage-Polenta Pie

PREP: 5 min; COOK: 19 min; BAKE: 25 min

6 SERVINGS

Any blend of frozen chunky-style vegetables works well in this recipe—use your favorite, or whatever you have on hand.

1 tube (16 ounces) refrigerated sun-dried tomato or plain polenta

1/2 pound bulk turkey Italian sausage

1 package (16 ounces) frozen potatoes, squash, zucchini, onion and red pepper

1 can (8 ounces) tomato sauce

1/4 cup shredded reduced-fat mozzarella cheese (1 ounce)

Heat oven to 425°. Spray pie plate, 9×1 1/4 inches, with nonstick cooking spray. Cut polenta into 1/4-inch slices; cut slices crosswise in half. Line bottom and side of pie plate with polenta, arranging slices around side with round edges up for scallop design. Bake 25 to 30 minutes or until golden brown.

Meanwhile, heat 10-inch skillet over medium-high heat. Cook sausage in skillet 8 to 10 minutes, stirring occasionally, until no longer pink; drain. Stir in vegetable mixture and tomato sauce; reduce heat to low. Cover and simmer 7 to 9 minutes, stirring occasionally, until vegetables are crisp-tender. Pour sausage mixture into polenta crust. Sprinkle with cheese. Cut into wedges.

1 Serving:		% Daily Value:	
Calories	205	Vitamin A	8%
Calories from fat	45	Vitamin C	8%
Fat, g	5	Calcium	4%
Saturated, g	2	Iron	14%
Cholesterol, mg	30	**Diet Exchanges:**	
Sodium, mg	960	2 starch/bread	
Carbohydrate, g	31	1 lean meat	
Dietary Fiber, g	5		
Protein, g	14		

Pasta with Beef, Broccoli and Tomatoes

PREP: 10 min; COOK: 15 min

6 SERVINGS

*Craving Oriental flavor? Just substitute soy sauce for
the Worcestershire sauce.*

**3 cups uncooked radiatore (nugget) pasta
(9 ounces)**

**3/4 pound beef boneless sirloin steak, cut
into 1/4-inch strips**

1/2 teaspoon pepper

**1 package (16 ounces) fresh or frozen
broccoli cuts (6 cups)**

**1 can (14 1/2 ounces) diced tomatoes with
roasted garlic, undrained**

**1 can (14 1/2 ounces) ready-to-serve beef
broth**

2 tablespoons cornstarch

2 tablespoons Worcestershire sauce

Cook and drain pasta as directed on package.
While pasta is cooking, spray 12-inch skillet with
nonstick cooking spray; heat over medium-high
heat. Add beef to skillet; sprinkle with pepper.
Cook 2 to 3 minutes, stirring frequently, until beef
is brown.

Stir in broccoli, tomatoes and broth; reduce heat
to low. Cover and simmer about 10 minutes, stirring occasionally, until broccoli is crisp-tender.
Mix cornstarch and Worcestershire sauce; stir into
beef mixture. Heat to boiling, stirring constantly.
Boil and stir 1 minute. Toss beef mixture and
pasta.

1 Serving:		% Daily Value:	
Calories	345	Vitamin A	18%
Calories from fat	25	Vitamin C	32%
Fat, g	3	Calcium	8%
Saturated, g	1	Iron	26%
Cholesterol, mg	25	**Diet Exchanges:**	
Sodium, mg	380	4 starch/bread	
Carbohydrate, g	61	1/2 lean meat	
Dietary Fiber, g	5		
Protein, g	23		

Salmon with Creamy Cucumber Sauce

PREP: 10 min; COOK: 13 min

4 SERVINGS

1 cup plain fat-free yogurt

1 tablespoon all-purpose flour

1 tablespoon chopped fresh or 1 teaspoon dried dill weed

1 teaspoon prepared horseradish

1 medium unpeeled cucumber, seeded and chopped (1 cup)

1 can (6 ounces) skinless, boneless pink salmon, drained and flaked

8 ounces uncooked spinach fettuccine

Mix yogurt and flour in 2-quart saucepan. Stir in dill weed and horseradish. Heat over low heat, stirring constantly, until hot (do not boil). Stir in cucumber and salmon; keep warm. Cook and drain fettuccine as directed on package. Serve sauce over fettuccine.

1 Serving:		% Daily Value:	
Calories	295	Vitamin A	2%
Calories from fat	45	Vitamin C	2%
Fat, g	5	Calcium	24%
Saturated, g	2	Iron	16%
Cholesterol, mg	75	**Diet Exchanges:**	
Sodium, mg	300	3 starch/bread	
Carbohydrate, g	45	1 lean meat	
Dietary Fiber, g	2		
Protein, g	20		

Capellini with Tomato-Shrimp Sauce

PREP: 10 min; COOK: 7 min

4 SERVINGS

Add a green salad a simple fruit dessert and you have a fast, and delicious, dinner.

6 ounces uncooked capellini (angel hair) pasta

1 teaspoon olive or vegetable oil

1/2 pound uncooked peeled deveined medium shrimp, thawed if frozen

1 can (15 ounces) Italian-style chunky tomato sauce

1/4 cup dry white wine or chicken broth

1/4 teaspoon crushed red pepper

1 tablespoon chopped fresh or 1 teaspoon dried basil leaves

Cook and drain pasta as directed on package. While pasta is cooking, heat oil in 12-inch skillet over medium-high heat. Cook shrimp in oil 1 to 2 minutes, stirring frequently, until shrimp are pink and firm.

Stir in tomato sauce, wine and red pepper; reduce heat to low. Simmer uncovered 5 minutes, stirring occasionally. Serve sauce over pasta. Sprinkle with basil.

1 Serving:		% Daily Value:	
Calories	225	Vitamin A	12%
Calories from fat	20	Vitamin C	12%
Fat, g	2	Calcium	4%
Saturated, g	0	Iron	18%
Cholesterol, mg	55	**Diet Exchanges:**	
Sodium, mg	710	2 starch/bread	
Carbohydrate, g	42	1/2 lean meat	
Dietary Fiber, g	3	2 vegetable	
Protein, g	13		

MALL WALKING

So the weather outside is frightful. It's too hot, humid, cold, snowy or icy. Or it could be there are no sidewalks to walk on or no safe area in which to walk. If so, join the recent craze of indoor mall walking at your favorite large shopping center.

Most large complexes open a designated set of outside doors before hours; individual stores are usually not open. Check with your local mall for walking hours and the mileage for one round around the perimeter of the mall. Of course you can walk around the mall anytime during open hours, but you may not be able to walk as quickly and may have to stop and start a number of times due to crowds.

If a walking group hasn't already been established, start your own with friends or neighbors. If window shopping doesn't suit you, try a radio or cassette headset to pass the time. Invest in shoes specifically designed for walking. If you've been walking for awhile and want to boost your workout, consider trying ankle or hand weights to increase the difficulty.

In addition to malls, schools or athletic facilities may offer walking; check with them and if they don't, request that they consider starting a program.

Scampi with Fettuccine

PREP: 10 min; COOK: 13 min

4 SERVINGS

6 ounces uncooked spinach fettuccine

1 pound uncooked peeled deveined medium shrimp, thawed if frozen

1 tablespoon chopped fresh or 1 1/2 teaspoons dried basil leaves

1 tablespoon chopped fresh parsley

2 tablespoons lemon juice

1/4 teaspoon salt

2 cloves garlic, finely chopped

1 medium green onion, thinly sliced (2 tablespoons)

Cook and drain fettuccine as directed on package. While fettuccine is cooking, spray 10-inch skillet with nonstick cooking spray; heat over medium heat. Cook remaining ingredients in skillet 2 to 3 minutes, stirring frequently, until shrimp are pink and firm; remove from heat. Add fettuccine to shrimp mixture; toss.

1 Serving:		% Daily Value:	
Calories	200	Vitamin A	4%
Calories from fat	20	Vitamin C	4%
Fat, g	2	Calcium	4%
Saturated, g	0	Iron	20%
Cholesterol, mg	145	**Diet Exchanges:**	
Sodium, mg	280	2 starch/bread	
Carbohydrate, g	29	1 lean meat	
Dietary Fiber, g	1		
Protein, g	17		

Scampi with Fettuccine

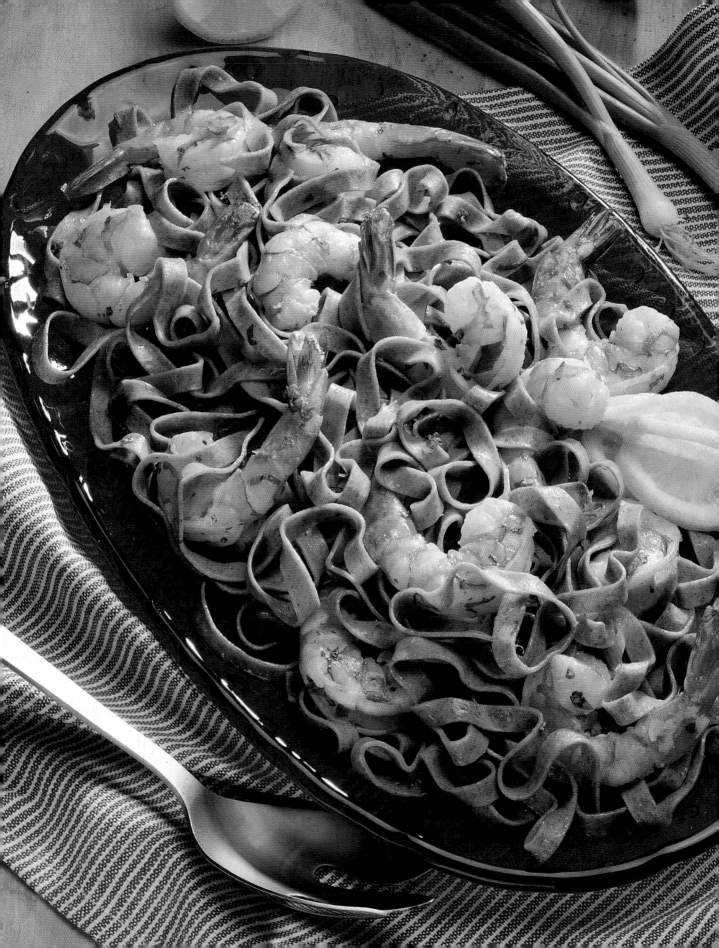

Easy Macaroni and Cheese

PREP: 10 min; COOK: 12 min

4 SERVINGS

1 package (7 ounces) small macaroni shells
  (2 cups)

1 tablespoon margarine or reduced-calorie
  spread

2 tablespoons all-purpose flour

1/4 teaspoon salt

1/4 teaspoon ground mustard (dry)

1/8 teaspoon pepper

1 cup skim milk

1 cup shredded reduced-fat Cheddar cheese
  (4 ounces)

1 medium green onion, sliced
  (2 tablespoons)

2 tablespoons chopped red bell pepper

Cook and drain macaroni as directed on package. While macaroni is cooking, melt margarine in 3-quart nonstick saucepan over low heat. Stir in flour, salt, mustard and pepper. Cook over low heat, stirring constantly, until margarine is absorbed; remove from heat. Gradually stir in milk. Heat to boiling, stirring constantly. Boil and stir 1 minute. Stir in cheese until melted.

Stir macaroni, onion and bell pepper into sauce. Cook, stirring constantly, until hot.

1 Serving:		% Daily Value:	
Calories	325	Vitamin A	12%
Calories from fat	80	Vitamin C	6%
Fat, g	9	Calcium	30%
Saturated, g	4	Iron	12%
Cholesterol, mg	15	**Diet Exchanges:**	
Sodium, mg	360	3 starch/bread	
Carbohydrate, g	46	1 high-fat meat	
Dietary Fiber, g	2		
Protein, g	17		

Mexican Macaroni and Cheese

PREP: 5 min; COOK: 15 min

4 SERVINGS

1 package (7 ounces) small macaroni shells
  (2 cups)

1/4 cup sliced ripe olives

1/2 cup fat-free half-and-half or skim milk

1/2 teaspoon salt

1 small red bell pepper, chopped (1/2 cup)

1 can (4 ounces) chopped green chilies,
  drained

4 slices fat-free American cheese (2 ounces)

Cook and drain macaroni as directed on package. Stir in remaining ingredients. Cook over low heat about 5 minutes, stirring occasionally, until cheese is melted and sauce is hot.

1 Serving:		% Daily Value:	
Calories	285	Vitamin A	10%
Calories from fat	20	Vitamin C	28%
Fat, g	2	Calcium	6%
Saturated, g	0	Iron	16%
Cholesterol, mg	0	**Diet Exchanges:**	
Sodium, mg	980	3 starch/bread	
Carbohydrate, g	56	1 vegetable	
Dietary Fiber, g	3	1/2 skim milk	
Protein, g	14		

Fettuccine with Creamy Tomato Sauce

PREP: 10 min; COOK: 13 min

5 SERVINGS

1 package (16 ounces) fettuccine

1 small onion, chopped (1/4 cup)

2 cloves garlic, finely chopped

2/3 cup reduced-fat ricotta cheese

1 tablespoon chopped fresh or 1 teaspoon dried basil leaves

1 tablespoon chopped fresh or 1 teaspoon freeze-dried chives

2 teaspoons sugar

1/8 teaspoon pepper

1 can (14 1/2 ounces) whole tomatoes, undrained

Cook and drain fettuccine as directed on package. While fettuccine is cooking, spray 3-quart saucepan with nonstick cooking spray; heat over medium-high heat. Cook onion and garlic in saucepan, stirring occasionally, until onion is crisp-tender. Stir in remaining ingredients, breaking up tomatoes.

Heat to boiling; reduce heat to low. Simmer uncovered about 5 minutes, stirring occasionally, until mixture thickens slightly. Add fettuccine to saucepan; toss with tomato sauce.

1 Serving:		% Daily Value:	
Calories	360	Vitamin A	8%
Calories from fat	35	Vitamin C	12%
Fat, g	4	Calcium	10%
Saturated, g	1	Iron	24%
Cholesterol, mg	80	**Diet Exchanges:**	
Sodium, mg	180	4 starch/bread	
Carbohydrate, g	68	1 vegetable	
Dietary Fiber, g	3		
Protein, g	16		

IS OLIVE OIL BETTER FOR YOU?

Fact: Eating a healthful diet means one that is similar to that of the Mediterranean region, with plenty of olive oil.

False: Olive oil may be helpful in reducing the level of "bad" low-density lipoprotein (LDL) cholesterol while maintaining the "good" high-density lipoprotein (HDL) cholesterol level in our blood. Thought to be the culprit in heart disease, LDL cholesterol contains most of the cholesterol found in the blood and is associated with making cholesterol available for cell structures, hormones and nerve coverings. LDL cholesterol also deposits cholesterol on artery walls. Conversely, HDL cholesterol helps to remove cholesterol from body tissues and blood and return it to the liver to be used again, thus this recycling process has earned the "good" cholesterol label.

Regardless of what experts tell us about this golden oil pressed from olives, it's still 100% fat, so it supplies the same amount of fat and calories as butter, margarine or other oils. Just the makeup of the fatty acids is different. So use olive oil sparingly, as you would any oil.

Garden-Fresh Primavera

PREP: 10 min; COOK: 13 min

4 SERVINGS

8 ounces uncooked linguine

1 cup 1-inch pieces green beans (4 ounces)

1 medium carrot, cut into 1/4-inch diagonal slices (1/2 cup)

1/2 medium green bell pepper, cut into 2×1/4-inch pieces

1 cup sliced mushrooms (3 ounces)

1 medium tomato, cut into 1-inch pieces (3/4 cup)

1 bottle (8 ounces) fat-free Caesar or creamy Italian dressing

Freshly ground pepper, if desired

Cook linguine as directed on package in 3-quart saucepan, adding green beans, carrot and bell pepper during last 3 minutes of cooking. While linguine is cooking, place mushrooms in colander. Drain linguine and vegetables in colander.

Return linguine and vegetables to saucepan. Add tomato and dressing; toss to coat. Cook over medium heat until hot. Serve with pepper.

1 Serving:		% Daily Value:	
Calories	265	Vitamin A	32%
Calories from fat	10	Vitamin C	14%
Fat, g	1	Calcium	4%
Saturated, g	0	Iron	16%
Cholesterol, mg	0	**Diet Exchanges:**	
Sodium, mg	620	3 starch/bread	
Carbohydrate, g	59	3 vegetable	
Dietary Fiber, g	4		
Protein, g	9		

Fettuccine Carbonara

PREP: 8 min; COOK: 13 min

6 SERVINGS

By using evaporated skimmed milk, fat-free cottage cheese and egg substitute, the calories in this carbonara have been cut in half, and it still keeps its wonderful flavor.

8 ounces uncooked fettuccine

3/4 cup evaporated skimmed milk

1/2 cup fat-free cottage cheese

1/4 cup fat-free cholesterol-free egg product

4 ounces Canadian-style bacon, chopped

1 cup frozen green peas

2 tablespoons grated fat-free Parmesan cheese

Freshly ground pepper

Cook and drain fettuccine as directed on package. Return fettuccine to saucepan.

Place skimmed milk, cottage cheese and egg product in blender or food processor. Cover and blend on medium speed about 1 minute or until smooth. Pour cottage cheese mixture over fettuccine. Add bacon, peas and Parmesan cheese. Cook over low heat 3 to 4 minutes, stirring constantly, until sauce is thickened. Sprinkle with pepper.

1 Serving:		% Daily Value:	
Calories	210	Vitamin A	6%
Calories from fat	25	Vitamin C	4%
Fat, g	3	Calcium	14%
Saturated, g	1	Iron	12%
Cholesterol, mg	45	**Diet Exchanges:**	
Sodium, mg	420	2 starch/bread	
Carbohydrate, g	32	1 lean meat	
Dietary Fiber, g	2		
Protein, g	16		

Fettuccine Carbonara

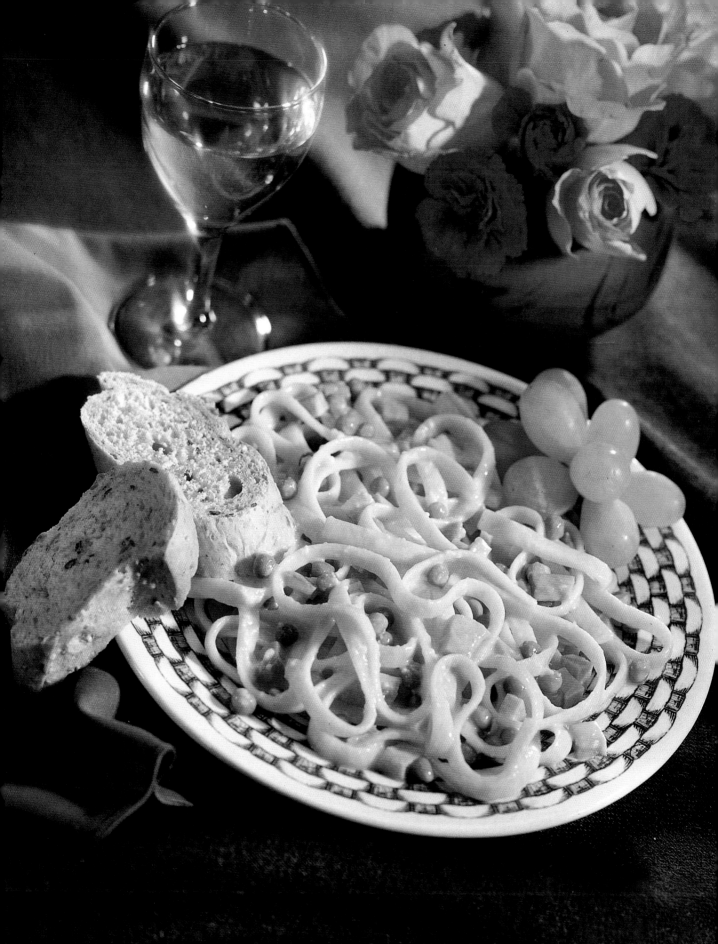

Spaghetti with Spicy Eggplant Sauce

PREP: 8 min; COOK: 18 min

5 SERVINGS

This spicy sauce provides an excellent contrast to whole wheat spaghetti.

8 ounces uncooked regular or whole wheat spaghetti

1 small eggplant (1 pound), peeled and cubed (3 cups)

1 can (14 1/2 ounces) Italian-style stewed tomatoes, undrained

1 can (8 ounces) no-salt-added tomato sauce

1/2 teaspoon crushed red pepper

2 tablespoons chopped fresh parsley or 2 teaspoons dried parsley flakes

Cook and drain spaghetti as directed on package. While spaghetti is cooking, heat eggplant, tomatoes, tomato sauce and red pepper to boiling in 10-inch skillet, stirring occasionally; reduce heat to low. Simmer uncovered about 15 minutes or until eggplant is tender. Stir in parsley. Serve over spaghetti.

1 Serving:		% Daily Value:	
Calories	215	Vitamin A	10%
Calories from fat	10	Vitamin C	18%
Fat, g	1	Calcium	4%
Saturated, g	0	Iron	16%
Cholesterol, mg	0	**Diet Exchanges:**	
Sodium, mg	150	3 starch/bread	
Carbohydrate, g	49	1 vegetable	
Dietary Fiber, g	5		
Protein, g	8		

Spaghetti with Spicy Eggplant Sauce

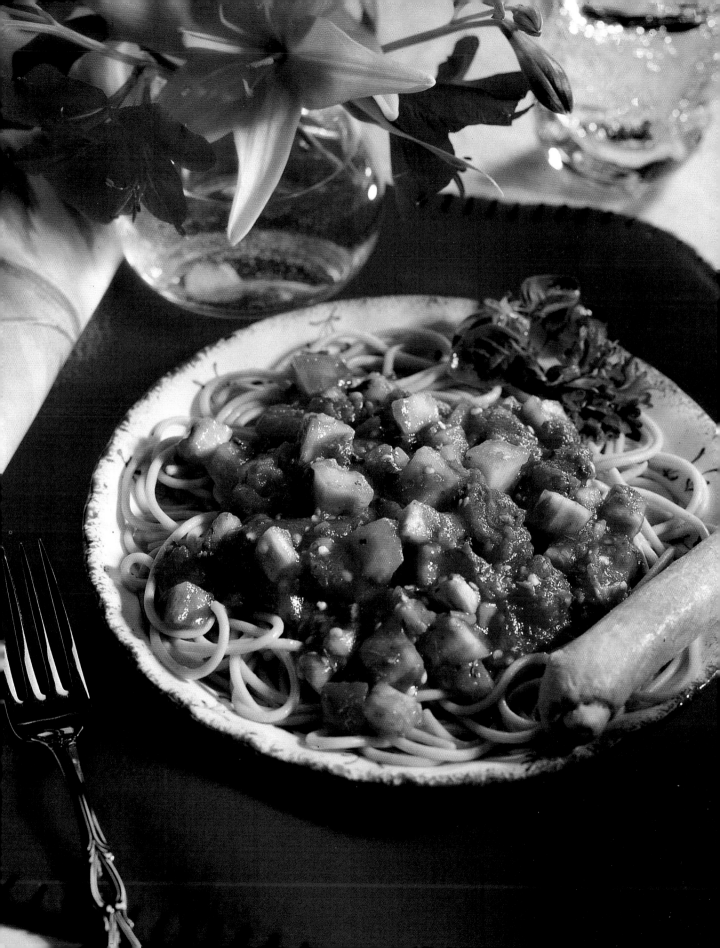

Spinach Fettuccine with Red Peppers

PREP: 10 min; COOK: 8 min

4 SERVINGS

Roasted red bell peppers add color and flavor to pasta, salads and sandwiches. The best part? Roasted peppers are also low in calories, fat and salt.

1 package (9 ounces) refrigerated spinach fettuccine

1 teaspoon olive or vegetable oil

3 cloves garlic, finely chopped

1 jar (7 1/4 ounces) roasted red bell peppers, drained and cut into 1/2-inch slices

4 ounces Canadian-style bacon, chopped

1/2 cup dry white wine or chicken broth

2 tablespoons chopped fresh parsley or 2 teaspoons dried parsley flakes

Cook and drain fettuccine as directed on package. While fettuccine is cooking, heat oil in 10-inch skillet over medium-high heat. Cook garlic in oil, stirring occasionally, until golden. Stir in bell peppers, bacon and wine. Heat to boiling; reduce heat to low. Simmer uncovered 5 minutes, stirring occasionally. Stir in parsley. Toss with fettuccine.

1 Serving:		% Daily Value:	
Calories	285	Vitamin A	16%
Calories from fat	55	Vitamin C	62%
Fat, g	6	Calcium	2%
Saturated, g	2	Iron	18%
Cholesterol, mg	70	**Diet Exchanges:**	
Sodium, mg	380	3 starch/bread	
Carbohydrate, g	46	1 lean meat	
Dietary Fiber, g	2		
Protein, g	14		

Portobello Stroganoff

PREP: 10 min; COOK: 10 min

4 SERVINGS

Portobello mushrooms have a texture similar to beef—they make a great substitute in this stroganoff.

4 cups uncooked cholesterol-free noodles (8 ounces)

1 tablespoon margarine

3/4 pound portobello mushrooms, cut into 2×1/2-inch strips

1 medium onion, chopped (1/2 cup)

1 clove garlic, chopped

3/4 cup beef broth

2 tablespoons ketchup

1/2 cup fat-free sour cream

Freshly ground pepper

Chopped fresh parsley, if desired

Cook and drain noodles as directed on package. While noodles are cooking, melt margarine in 12-inch skillet over medium heat. Cook mushrooms, onion and garlic in margarine, stirring occasionally, until mushrooms are brown and tender. Stir in broth and ketchup. Cook 5 minutes, stirring occasionally. Stir in sour cream. Serve over noodles. Sprinkle with pepper and parsley.

1 Serving:		% Daily Value:	
Calories	215	Vitamin A	10%
Calories from fat	25	Vitamin C	4%
Fat, g	3	Calcium	10%
Saturated, g	0	Iron	16%
Cholesterol, mg	0	**Diet Exchanges:**	
Sodium, mg	280	2 starch/bread	
Carbohydrate, g	40	2 vegetable	
Dietary Fiber, g	3		
Protein, g	10		

Meatless Meatball Pizza

PREP: 10 min; BAKE: 20 min

6 SERVINGS

This pizza tastes just like traditional Italian sausage pizza!

1 package (10 ounces) thin Italian bread shell or ready-to-serve pizza crust (12 to 14 inches in diameter)

2 frozen soybean-based vegetable burgers, thawed

1 tablespoon grated fat-free Parmesan cheese

1/2 teaspoon Italian seasoning, crumbled

3/4 cup pizza sauce

2 tablespoons sliced ripe olives

2 cups shredded reduced-fat mozzarella cheese (4 ounces)

Heat oven to 425°. Place bread shell on ungreased cookie sheet. Mix burgers, Parmesan cheese and Italian seasoning. Shape into 1/2-inch balls. Spread pizza sauce over bread shell. Top with burger balls and olives. Sprinkle with mozzarella cheese. Bake 18 to 20 minutes or until cheese is melted and light golden brown.

1 Serving:		% Daily Value:	
Calories	310	Vitamin A	16%
Calories from fat	70	Vitamin C	4%
Fat, g	8	Calcium	26%
Saturated, g	2	Iron	16%
Cholesterol, mg	0	**Diet Exchanges:**	
Sodium, mg	910	3 starch/bread	
Carbohydrate, g	49	1 lean meat	
Dietary Fiber, g	5	1 vegetable	
Protein, g	16		

Hawaiian Pizza

PREP: 8 min; BAKE: 10 min

6 SERVINGS

1 package (10 ounces) thin Italian bread shell or ready-to-serve pizza crust (12 to 14 inches in diameter)

1 can (8 ounces) tomato sauce

2 cups cubed cooked chicken breast

1 can (8 ounces) pineapple tidbits, well drained

1 cup shredded reduced-fat mozzarella cheese (4 ounces)

Heat oven to 400°. Place bread shell on ungreased cookie sheet. Spread tomato sauce over bread shell. Top with chicken and pineapple. Sprinkle with cheese. Bake 8 to 10 minutes or until pizza is hot and cheese is melted.

1 Serving:		% Daily Value:	
Calories	315	Vitamin A	10%
Calories from fat	45	Vitamin C	6%
Fat, g	5	Calcium	12%
Saturated, g	2	Iron	10%
Cholesterol, mg	35	**Diet Exchanges:**	
Sodium, mg	740	2 starch/bread	
Carbohydrate, g	48	2 lean meat	
Dietary Fiber, g	3	1 fruit	
Protein, g	22		

Pizza Primavera

PREP: 10 min; COOK: 5 min; BAKE: 17 min

6 SERVINGS

We cooked the vegetables in fat-free Italian dressing instead of oil to reduce the fat, but keep the flavor.

1 loaf (1 pound) frozen honey-wheat or white bread dough, thawed

1/4 cup fat-free Italian dressing

1/2 pound asparagus, cut into 1-inch pieces

2 medium carrots, sliced (1 cup)

1 cup small broccoli flowerets

3 roma (plum) tomatoes, thinly sliced

1 cup shredded reduced-fat mozzarella cheese (4 ounces)

Heat oven to 450°. Spray cookie sheet with nonstick cooking spray. Pat or roll dough into 12-inch circle on cookie sheet. Prick dough thoroughly with fork. Bake 8 minutes (if dough puffs during baking, flatten with spoon).

Heat dressing to boiling in 10-inch nonstick skillet. Stir in asparagus, carrots and broccoli. Heat to boiling; reduce heat to medium. Cover and cook 3 to 4 minutes or until vegetables are crisp-tender.

Place tomato slices on partially baked crust. Spread vegetable mixture evenly over tomatoes. Sprinkle with cheese. Bake 7 to 9 minutes or until cheese is melted and crust is golden brown.

1 Serving:		% Daily Value:	
Calories	265	Vitamin A	50%
Calories from fat	55	Vitamin C	24%
Fat, g	6	Calcium	20%
Saturated, g	2	Iron	16%
Cholesterol, mg	0	**Diet Exchanges:**	
Sodium, mg	630	3 starch/bread	
Carbohydrate, g	48	1 vegetable	
Dietary Fiber, g	5		
Protein, g	10		

Pizza Primavera

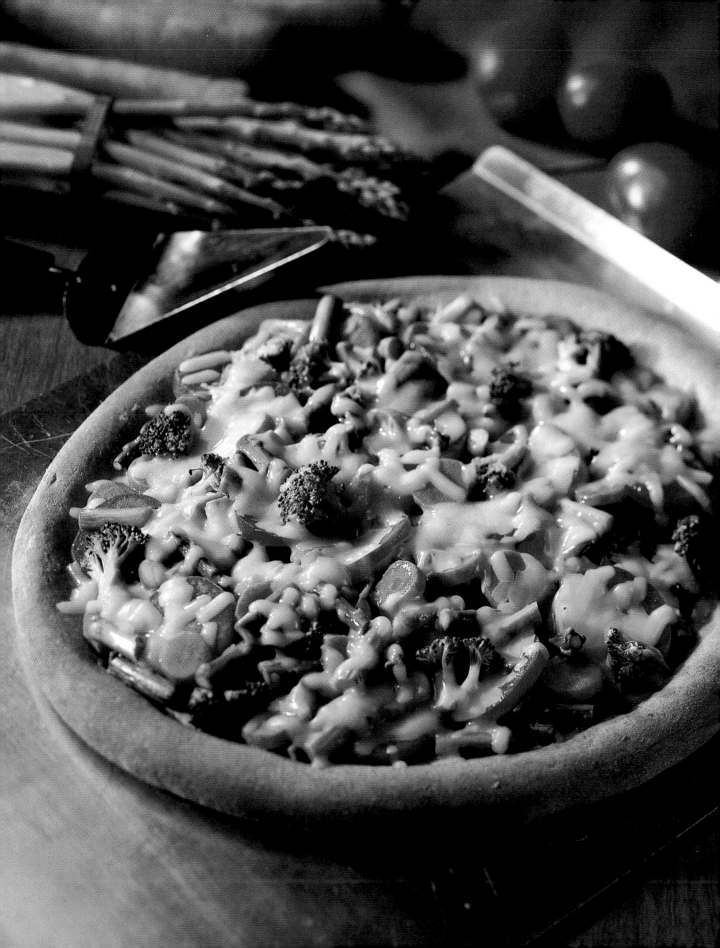

Roasted-Vegetable Pizza

PREP: 15 min; BAKE: 40 min

8 SERVINGS

The vegetables for this recipe can easily be prepared ahead of time and refrigerated until you make the pizza.

1 medium bell pepper, cut lengthwise into eighths

1 medium zucchini, cut into 1/4-inch slices

1/2 small eggplant (1/2 pound), cut into 1/4-inch slices

1 package (8 ounces) fresh portobello mushrooms, cut into 1/2-inch slices

2 tablespoons roasted garlic-flavored or regular vegetable oil

1/2 teaspoon salt

1/4 teaspoon pepper

1 package (10 ounces) thin Italian bread shell or ready-to-serve pizza crust (12 to 14 inches in diameter)

1/2 cup shredded reduced-fat mozzarella cheese (2 ounces)

Heat oven to 400°. Spray jelly roll pan 15 1/2×10 1/2×1 inch, with nonstick cooking spray. Place bell pepper, zucchini, eggplant and mushrooms in single layer in pan. Brush with oil. Sprinkle with salt and pepper. Bake 25 to 30 minutes, turning vegetables once, until edges of vegetables are light brown.

Place bread shell on ungreased cookie sheet. Top with vegetables. Sprinkle with cheese. Bake 8 to 10 minutes or until cheese is melted.

1 Serving:		% Daily Value:	
Calories	195	Vitamin A	4%
Calories from fat	55	Vitamin C	10%
Fat, g	6	Calcium	4%
Saturated, g	1	Iron	8%
Cholesterol, mg	0	**Diet Exchanges:**	
Sodium, mg	460	2 starch/bread	
Carbohydrate, g	32	1 fat	
Dietary Fiber, g	3		
Protein, g	6		

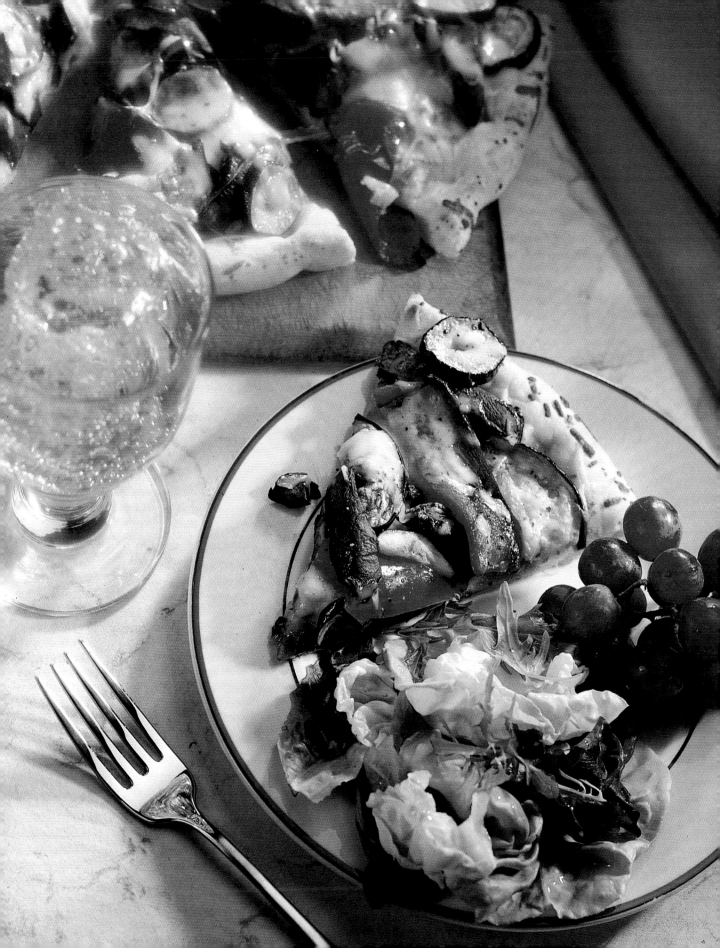

Wild Mushroom Pizza

PREP: 15 min; COOK: 6 min; BAKE: 8 min

8 SERVINGS

Wild mushrooms give this pizza an exotic flavor—use any combination that you like. If wild mushrooms are unavailable, use regular domestic white mushrooms.

1 tablespoon olive or vegetable oil

1 pound assorted fresh mushrooms (such as morel, oyster and shiitake), sliced (6 cups)

1 medium onion, chopped (1/2 cup)

2 cloves garlic, finely chopped

2 tablespoons chopped fresh parsley

1 package (10 ounces) thin Italian bread shell or ready-to-serve pizza crust (12 to 14 inches in diameter)

1/2 cup finely shredded Parmesan cheese

Heat oven to 450°. Heat oil in 12-inch nonstick skillet over high heat. Cook mushrooms, onion and garlic in oil about 5 minutes, stirring frequently or until onion is crisp-tender. Stir in parsley. Place bread shell on ungreased cookie sheet. Top with mushroom mixture. Sprinkle with cheese. Bake 8 to 10 minutes or until cheese is melted.

1 Serving:		% Daily Value:	
Calories	240	Vitamin A	0%
Calories from fat	55	Vitamin C	4%
Fat, g	6	Calcium	10%
Saturated, g	2	Iron	6%
Cholesterol, mg	5	**Diet Exchanges:**	
Sodium, mg	470	2 starch/bread	
Carbohydrate, g	40	2 vegetable	
Dietary Fiber, g	4	1 fat	
Protein, g	10		

Easy Vegetable Pizza

PREP: 8 min; COOK: 8 min; BAKE: 10 min

4 SERVINGS

1 package (10 ounces) thin Italian bread shell or ready-to-serve pizza crust (12 to 14 inches in diameter)

2/3 cup pizza sauce

1 teaspoon olive or vegetable oil

1 clove garlic, finely chopped

1 small onion, chopped (1/4 cup)

2 cups broccoli slaw or shredded carrot and zucchini

2/3 cup shredded reduced-fat mozzarella cheese

2 tablespoons grated fat-free Parmesan cheese

Heat oven to 450°. Place bread shell on cookie sheet. Spread pizza sauce evenly over bread shell.

Heat oil in 8-inch skillet over medium heat. Cook garlic and onion in oil about 2 minutes, stirring occasionally, until onion is crisp-tender. Stir in broccoli slaw. Cook 5 to 6 minutes, stirring occasionally, until broccoli is crisp-tender, adding up to 2 tablespoons water if necessary to prevent sticking.

Spoon vegetable mixture evenly over pizza sauce. Sprinkle with cheeses. Bake about 10 minutes or until cheese is melted.

1 Serving:		% Daily Value:	
Calories	335	Vitamin A	60%
Calories from fat	45	Vitamin C	12%
Fat, g	5	Calcium	18%
Saturated, g	1	Iron	4%
Cholesterol, mg	2	**Diet Exchanges:**	
Sodium, mg	890	4 starch/bread	
Carbohydrate, g	65	1 vegetable	
Dietary Fiber, g	5		
Protein, g	12		

Fireworks Pizza

PREP: 5 min; BAKE: 12 min

8 SERVINGS

Giardiniera vegetable mix is sold in the supermarket section with the pickles. The mixture contains carrots, broccoli, cauliflower and other vegetables. Pepperoncini peppers are located in the same section, too.

1 package (10 ounces) thin Italian bread shell or ready-to-serve pizza crust (12 to 14 inches in diameter)

1 jar (12 ounces) giardiniera vegetable mix, well drained

1 tablespoon chopped drained pepperoncini peppers

3/4 cup crumbled feta cheese

2 teaspoons chopped fresh parsley or 1 teaspoon dried parsley flakes

Heat oven to 400°. Place bread shell on ungreased cookie sheet. Mix vegetable mix and peppers; spread evenly over bread shell. Sprinkle with cheese and parsley. Bake 10 to 12 minutes or until cheese is melted and bubbly.

1 Serving:		% Daily Value:	
Calories	190	Vitamin A	2%
Calories from fat	35	Vitamin C	2%
Fat, g	4	Calcium	8%
Saturated, g	2	Iron	0%
Cholesterol, mg	15	**Diet Exchanges:**	
Sodium, mg	420	2 starch/bread	
Carbohydrate, g	34	1 vegetable	
Dietary Fiber, g	2		
Protein, g	6		

Pita Pizzas

PREP: 12 min; COOK: 6 min; BAKE: 7 min

4 SERVINGS

4 whole wheat pita breads (6 inches in diameter)

1 can (15 to 16 ounces) great northern beans, drained and 1/4 cup liquid reserved

1 small onion, chopped (1/4 cup)

1 clove garlic, finely chopped

2 tablespoons chopped fresh or 2 teaspoons dried basil leaves

1 large tomato, seeded and coarsely chopped (1 cup)

1 large green bell pepper, coarsely chopped (1 1/2 cups)

1 cup shredded reduced-fat mozzarella cheese (4 ounces)

Heat oven to 425°. Split each pita bread around edge with knife to make 2 rounds. Place in ungreased jelly roll pan, 15 1/2×10 1/2×1 inch. Bake about 5 minutes or just until crisp.

Heat reserved bean liquid to boiling in 10-inch nonstick skillet. Cook onion and garlic in bean liquid over medium heat 5 minutes, stirring occasionally. Stir in beans; heat through.

Mash bean mixture until almost smooth; stir in basil. Spread about 2 tablespoons bean mixture on each pita bread half. Top with tomato and bell pepper. Sprinkle with cheese. Bake in jelly roll pan 5 to 7 minutes or until cheese is melted.

1 Serving:		% Daily Value:	
Calories	345	Vitamin A	8%
Calories from fat	65	Vitamin C	26%
Fat, g	7	Calcium	30%
Saturated, g	4	Iron	28%
Cholesterol, mg	15	**Diet Exchanges:**	
Sodium, mg	660	3 starch/bread	
Carbohydrate, g	59	1 lean meat	
Dietary Fiber, g	10	1 vegetable	
Protein, g	22	1/2 skim milk	

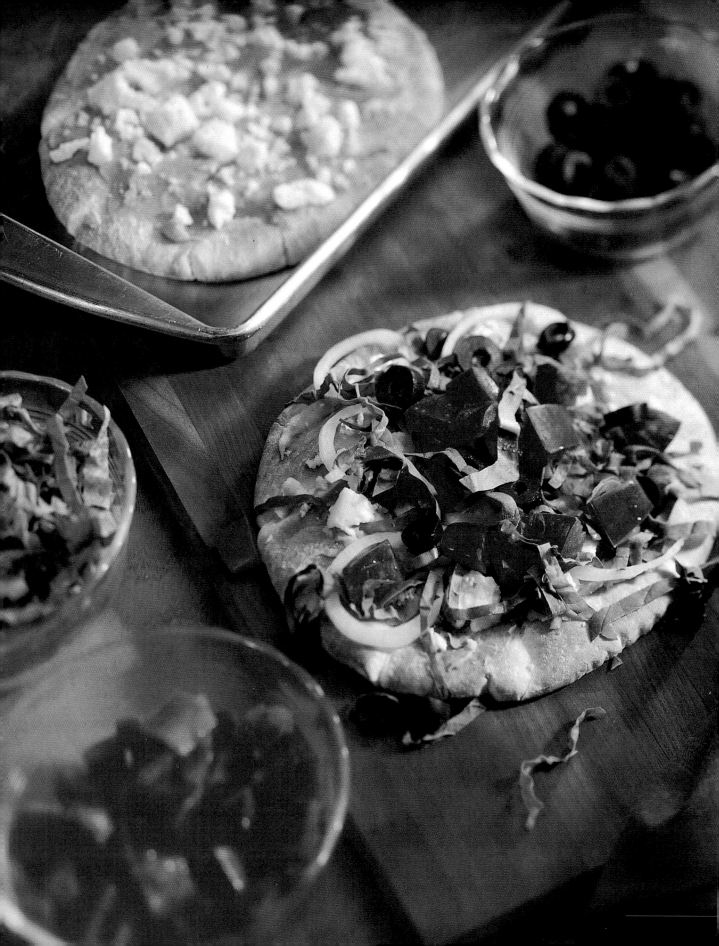

Middle Eastern Pita Pizzas

PREP: 10 min; BAKE: 10 min

4 SERVINGS

Hummus is a thick Middle Eastern sauce made from mashed garbanzo beans and tahini and is seasoned with lemon juice, garlic and olive oil. Prepared hummus is available in the refrigerated deli section of your supermarket.

4 fat-free pita breads (6 inches in diameter)

1/2 cup roasted-garlic flavor or regular hummus

1 cup crumbled feta cheese (4 ounces)

1 small onion, sliced

2 cups shredded spinach

1 large tomato, seeded and chopped (1 cup)

1/4 cup sliced ripe olives

Heat oven to 400°. Place pita breads in jelly roll pan, 15 1/2×10 1/2×1 inch. Spread hummus on each pita bread; sprinkle with cheese. Bake 8 to 10 minutes or until cheese is melted. Sprinkle each pizza with onion, spinach, tomato and olives.

1 Serving:		% Daily Value:	
Calories	305	Vitamin A	24%
Calories from fat	80	Vitamin C	16%
Fat, g	9	Calcium	30%
Saturated, g	6	Iron	18%
Cholesterol, mg	35	**Diet Exchanges:**	
Sodium, mg	840	3 starch/bread	
Carbohydrate, g	46	1 1/2 fat	
Dietary Fiber, g	3		
Protein, g	13		

Middle Eastern Pita Pizzas

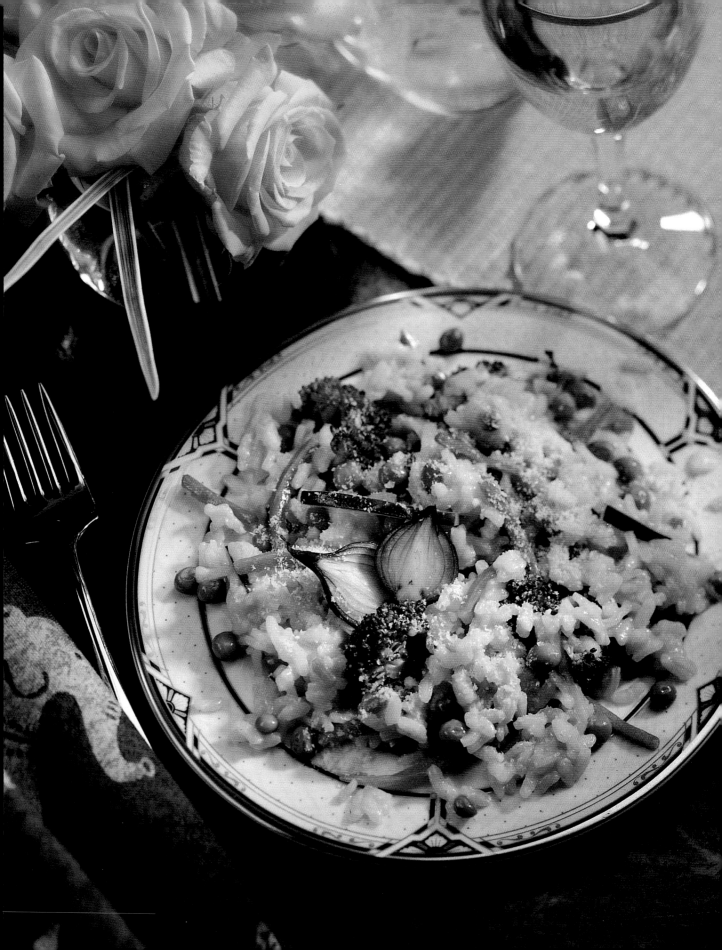

8

Rice, Beans and Grain Main Dishes

Risotto Primavera
(page 176)

Risotto Primavera

PREP: 12 min; COOK: 30 min

4 SERVINGS

2 teaspoons olive or vegetable oil

1 medium onion, chopped (1/2 cup)

2 small carrots, cut into julienne strips (1 cup)

1 cup uncooked Arborio or regular medium-grain white rice

2 cans (14 1/2 ounces each) ready-to-serve fat-free reduced-sodium chicken broth

2 cups broccoli flowerets

1 cup frozen green peas

2 small zucchini, cut into julienne strips (1 cup)

3 tablespoons grated fat-free Parmesan cheese

Heat oil in 3-quart nonstick saucepan over medium-high heat. Cook onion and carrot in oil, stirring frequently, until crisp-tender. Stir in rice. Cook, stirring frequently, until rice begins to brown.

Pour 1/2 cup of the broth over rice mixture. Cook uncovered, stirring occasionally, until liquid is absorbed. Continue cooking 15 to 20 minutes, adding broth 1/2 cup at a time and stirring occasionally, until rice is tender and creamy; add broccoli, peas and zucchini with the last addition of broth. Sprinkle with cheese.

1 Serving:		% Daily Value:	
Calories	250	Vitamin A	24%
Calories from fat	40	Vitamin C	20%
Fat, g	4	Calcium	8%
Saturated, g	0	Iron	16%
Cholesterol, mg	0	**Diet Exchanges:**	
Sodium, mg	460	2 starch/bread	
Carbohydrate, g	50	4 vegetable	
Dietary Fiber, g	4		
Protein, g	8		

Creamy Corn and Garlic Risotto

PREP: 5 min; COOK: 27 min

4 SERVINGS

Arborio rice, a specialty of Italy, creates the creamiest risotto, but you can substitute any medium-grain white rice in this recipe.

3 3/4 cups ready-to-serve fat-free reduced-sodium chicken broth

4 cloves garlic, finely chopped

1 cup uncooked Arborio or regular medium-grain white rice

3 cups frozen whole kernel corn

1/2 cup grated fat-free Parmesan cheese

1/3 cup shredded reduced-fat mozzarella cheese

1/4 cup chopped fresh parsley

Heat 1/3 cup of the broth to boiling in 10-inch skillet. Cook garlic in broth 1 minute, stirring occasionally. Stir in rice and corn. Cook 1 minute, stirring occasionally.

Stir in remaining broth; heat to boiling. Reduce heat to medium. Continue cooking, uncovered, 15 to 20 minutes, stirring occasionally, until rice is tender and creamy; remove from heat. Stir in cheeses and parsley.

1 Serving:		% Daily Value:	
Calories	330	Vitamin A	8%
Calories from fat	20	Vitamin C	8%
Fat, g	2	Calcium	22%
Saturated, g	0	Iron	14%
Cholesterol, mg	10	**Diet Exchanges:**	
Sodium, mg	660	4 starch/bread	
Carbohydrate, g	67	1 vegetable	
Dietary Fiber, g	3		
Protein, g	14		

WHAT DOES AEROBIC MEAN?

The word *aerobic* has been used a number of times in this book. When people hear the word *aerobic*, they immediately think of aerobic dance classes, but the classification of aerobic activities is much broader than that. Aerobic basically means "with oxygen," whereas, the term *anaerobic* means "without oxygen." Your body needs to take in oxygen to fuel your working muscles.

What is aerobic activity?

- It demands oxygen.
- It elevates your heart rate.
- It uses large muscle groups for an extended period of time (fifteen to sixty minutes).

Examples of aerobic activities are walking, running, cross-country skiing, swimming, in-line skating, biking and many more! Choose activities you enjoy because to make it beneficial, you need to make a commitment to do it at least three to five times each week.

Artichoke Hearts in Tomato Rice

PREP: 5 min; COOK: 12 min

6 SERVINGS

3 cups uncooked instant rice

1/2 teaspoon salt

6 medium green onions, chopped (1/3 cup)

2 cans (16 ounces each) stewed tomatoes, undrained

2 cans (14 ounces each) artichoke hearts, undrained

Mix all ingredients in 12-inch skillet. Heat to boiling, stirring frequently; reduce heat to low. Cover and simmer about 10 minutes or until rice is tender.

1 Serving:		% Daily Value:	
Calories	300	Vitamin A	12%
Calories from fat	20	Vitamin C	32%
Fat, g	2	Calcium	12%
Saturated, g	0	Iron	24%
Cholesterol, mg	0	**Diet Exchanges:**	
Sodium, mg	840	4 starch/bread	
Carbohydrate, g	70	2 vegetable	
Dietary Fiber, g	10		
Protein, g	10		

Southern Stir-Fry

PREP: 5 min; COOK: 8 min

4 SERVINGS

2 cups cold cooked white rice

1 cup frozen whole kernel corn

1 1/2 teaspoons chopped fresh or 1/2 teaspoon dried thyme leaves

1/4 teaspoon salt

1/4 teaspoon garlic powder

1/8 teaspoon ground red pepper (cayenne)

1 can (15 to 16 ounces) black-eyed peas, rinsed and drained

2 cups firmly packed spinach leaves

Spray 12-inch nonstick skillet with nonstick cooking spray; heat over medium-high heat. Cook all ingredients except spinach in skillet, stirring occasionally, until hot. Stir in spinach. Cook until spinach begins to wilt.

1 Serving:		% Daily Value:	
Calories	220	Vitamin A	24%
Calories from fat	10	Vitamin C	8%
Fat, g	1	Calcium	6%
Saturated, g	0	Iron	22%
Cholesterol, mg	0	**Diet Exchanges:**	
Sodium, mg	390	3 starch/bread	
Carbohydrate, g	50	1 vegetable	
Dietary Fiber, g	8		
Protein, g	11		

Wild Rice and Vegetable Stir-Fry

PREP: 8 min; COOK: 12 min

4 SERVINGS

1/4 cup dry white wine or ready-to-serve fat-free reduced-sodium chicken broth

1 tablespoon olive or vegetable oil

1 large onion, chopped (1 cup)

3 cloves garlic, finely chopped

3 cups frozen sliced bell peppers (from 16-ounce package)

2 cups cooked wild rice

1/4 cup chopped fresh parsley

1/4 cup reduced-sodium soy sauce

1 Serving:		% Daily Value:	
Calories	150	Vitamin A	6%
Calories from fat	35	Vitamin C	62%
Fat, g	4	Calcium	2%
Saturated, g	1	Iron	8%
Cholesterol, mg	0	**Diet Exchanges:**	
Sodium, mg	610	1 starch/bread	
Carbohydrate, g	28	2 vegetable	
Dietary Fiber, g	4	1/2 fat	
Protein, g	5		

Heat wine and oil to boiling in 10-inch skillet over medium-high heat. Cook onion and garlic in wine and oil about 8 minutes, stirring frequently, until onion is tender. Add bell peppers and wild rice; stir-fry 2 minutes. Add parsley and soy sauce; heat through.

Basque Vegetarian Paella

PREP: 8 min; COOK: 26 min

4 SERVINGS

Canned artichoke hearts and a mix of frozen vegetables make this traditional Spanish stew a fast, colorful dish.

2 large onions, chopped (2 cups)

5 cloves garlic, finely chopped

1 cup uncooked basmati or regular long grain rice

1 can (14 ounces) quartered artichoke hearts, drained

1 package (16 ounces) cauliflower, carrots and snow pea pods, thawed

1 cup frozen sliced bell peppers (from 16-ounce package)

2 cups dry white wine or ready-to-serve fat-free reduced-sodium chicken broth

1 teaspoon salt

Spray 10-inch nonstick skillet with nonstick cooking spray; heat over medium-high heat. Cook onions and garlic in skillet about 8 minutes, stirring occasionally, until onions are tender.

Stir in rice and artichoke hearts. Cook 3 minutes, stirring occasionally. Stir in wine and salt. Heat to boiling; reduce heat to low. Cover and simmer about 10 minutes. Stir in vegetables. Cover and cook 5 minutes or until liquid is absorbed.

1 Serving:		% Daily Value:	
Calories	295	Vitamin A	84%
Calories from fat	10	Vitamin C	36%
Fat, g	1	Calcium	10%
Saturated, g	0	Iron	26%
Cholesterol, mg	0	**Diet Exchanges:**	
Sodium, mg	920	4 starch/bread	
Carbohydrate, g	71	2 vegetable	
Dietary Fiber, g	11		
Protein, g	11		

Basque Vegetarian Paella

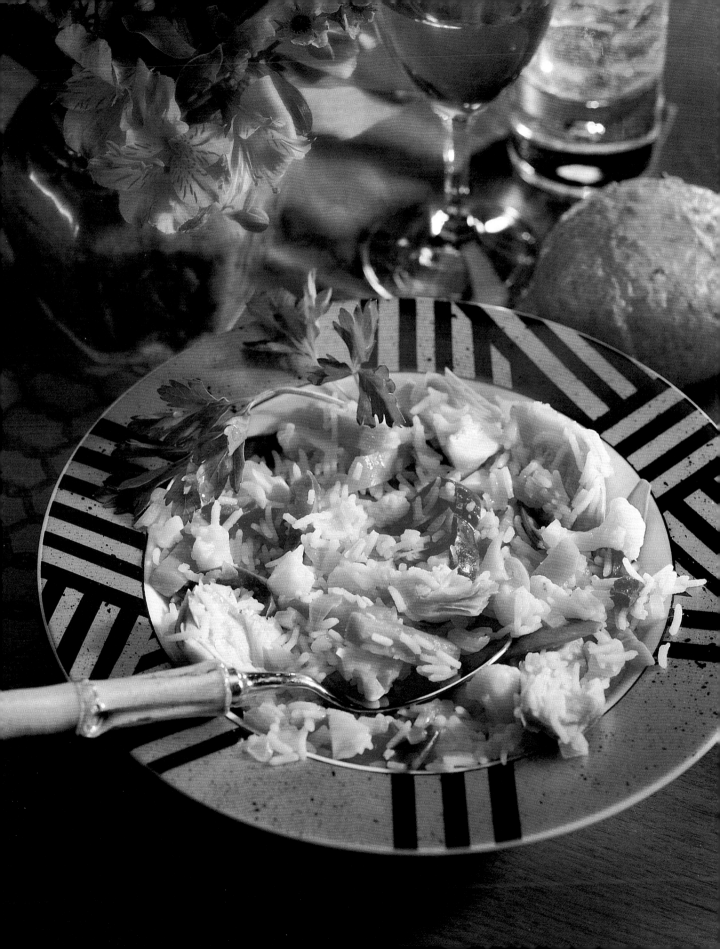

Mexican Rice and Bean Bake

PREP: 10 min; BAKE: 35 min; STAND: 5 min

6 SERVINGS

2 cups cooked brown or white rice

1/4 cup fat-free cholesterol-free egg product

1 1/2 cups picante sauce or salsa

1 cup shredded reduced-fat Cheddar cheese (4 ounces)

1 teaspoon chili powder

1 can (15 to 16 ounces) pinto beans, rinsed and drained

Heat oven to 350°. Spray square baking dish, 8 × 8 × 2 inches, with nonstick cooking spray. Mix rice, egg product, 1/2 cup of the picante sauce, 1/2 cup of the cheese and the chili powder; press in bottom of baking dish.

Mix beans and remaining 1 cup picante sauce; spoon over rice mixture. Sprinkle with remaining 1/2 cup cheese. Bake uncovered 30 to 35 minutes or until cheese is melted and bubbly. Let stand 5 minutes before serving.

1 Serving:		% Daily Value:	
Calories	195	Vitamin A	8%
Calories from fat	35	Vitamin C	12%
Fat, g	4	Calcium	20%
Saturated, g	2	Iron	14%
Cholesterol, mg	10	**Diet Exchanges:**	
Sodium, mg	440	2 starch/bread	
Carbohydrate, g	35	1 vegetable	
Dietary Fiber, g	8		
Protein, g	13		

Lentil and Brown Rice Casserole

PREP: 10 min; BAKE: 1 1/2 hr

6 SERVINGS

3/4 cup dried lentils, sorted and rinsed

1/2 cup uncooked brown rice

2 cans (10 1/2 ounces each) ready-to-serve low-sodium chicken broth

1/4 teaspoon salt

1 cup shredded reduced-fat Cheddar cheese (4 ounces)

1 package (16 ounces) frozen cut green beans or broccoli cuts, thawed and drained

Heat oven to 375°. Mix lentils, rice, broth, salt and 3/4 cup of the cheese in 2-quart casserole. Cover and bake 1 hour.

Stir in green beans. Cover and bake about 30 minutes or until liquid is absorbed and rice is tender. Sprinkle with remaining 1/4 cup cheese.

1 Serving:		% Daily Value:	
Calories	185	Vitamin A	4%
Calories from fat	35	Vitamin C	2%
Fat, g	4	Calcium	18%
Saturated, g	2	Iron	18%
Cholesterol, mg	10	**Diet Exchanges:**	
Sodium, mg	380	1 starch/bread	
Carbohydrate, g	31	2 vegetable	
Dietary Fiber, g	8	1/2 skim milk	
Protein, g	14		

Black Bean and Corn Salad

PREP: 10 min

4 SERVINGS

Rinsing beans before using removes some of the salt, which is particularly helpful if you're watching your sodium intake.

1 can (15 ounces) black beans, rinsed and drained

1 cup frozen whole kernel corn, thawed

1/4 cup chopped fresh cilantro or parsley

1/4 cup salsa

2 tablespoons lime juice

1/4 teaspoon salt

4 lettuce leaves

Mix all ingredients except lettuce. Place lettuce leaf on each of 4 salad plates. Top with bean mixture.

1 Serving:		% Daily Value:	
Calories	150	Vitamin A	6%
Calories from fat	10	Vitamin C	8%
Fat, g	1	Calcium	8%
Saturated, g	0	Iron	14%
Cholesterol, mg	0	**Diet Exchanges:**	
Sodium, mg	410	2 starch/bread	
Carbohydrate, g	34	1 vegetable	
Dietary Fiber, g	8		
Protein, g	9		

New Mexican Black Bean Burritos

PREP: 8 min; COOK: 7 min

4 SERVINGS

Chipotle chilies, which are smoked jalapeño chilies, make this a spicy dish. Garnish the burritos with extra chopped tomato, cilantro and fat-free yogurt.

1 large onion, chopped (1 cup)

6 cloves garlic, finely chopped

1 can (15 ounces) black beans, rinsed, drained and mashed

1 to 2 teaspoons finely chopped chipotle chilies in adobo sauce, drained

4 fat-free flour tortillas (6 to 8 inches in diameter)

1/2 cup shredded reduced-fat mozzarella cheese (2 ounces)

1 large tomato, chopped (1 cup)

Spray 10-inch nonstick skillet with nonstick cooking spray; heat over medium-high heat. Cook onion and garlic in skillet about 5 minutes, stirring occasionally, until onion is tender but not brown. Stir in beans and chilies; cook until hot. Place one-fourth of the bean mixture on center of each tortilla. Top with cheese and tomato.

Fold one end of tortilla up about 1 inch over filling; fold right and left sides over folded end, overlapping. Fold remaining end down. Place seam side down on serving platter or plate.

1 Serving:		% Daily Value:	
Calories	235	Vitamin A	8%
Calories from fat	20	Vitamin C	10%
Fat, g	2	Calcium	20%
Saturated, g	0	Iron	18%
Cholesterol, mg	0	**Diet Exchanges:**	
Sodium, mg	450	3 starch/bread	
Carbohydrate, g	49	1 vegetable	
Dietary Fiber, g	6		
Protein, g	11		

Sweet Potatoes and Black Beans

PREP: 10 min; COOK: 20 min

5 SERVINGS

3 medium sweet potatoes, peeled and cut into 3/4-inch cubes (3 cups)

3/4 cup orange juice

2 teaspoons cornstarch

1/2 teaspoon ground coriander

1/2 teaspoon ground allspice

1/2 teaspoon grated gingerroot or 1/4 teaspoon ground ginger

1/4 teaspoon ground cumin

1 can (15 ounces) black beans, rinsed and drained

1 cup cooked rice

Place sweet potatoes in 2-quart saucepan; add enough water just to cover sweet potatoes. Heat to boiling; reduce heat to low. Cover and simmer 10 to 12 minutes or until tender; drain and set aside.

Mix remaining ingredients except beans and rice in same saucepan. Heat to boiling. Boil about 1 minute, stirring constantly, until thickened. Stir in sweet potatoes, beans and rice. Cook about 2 minutes or until hot.

1 Serving:		% Daily Value:	
Calories	215	Vitamin A	100%
Calories from fat	10	Vitamin C	26%
Fat, g	1	Calcium	8%
Saturated, g	0	Iron	14%
Cholesterol, mg	0	**Diet Exchanges:**	
Sodium, mg	180	3 starch/bread	
Carbohydrate, g	50	1 vegetable	
Dietary Fiber, g	7		
Protein, g	8		

Savory Black-Eyed Peas

PREP: 10 min; COOK: 15 min

4 SERVINGS

Sprinkle each serving with imitation bacon bits to add the traditional smokey flavor without the fat.

1 cup ready-to-serve fat-free reduced-sodium chicken broth

3 medium carrots, thinly sliced (1 1/2 cups)

2 medium stalks celery, sliced (1 cup)

1 large onion, chopped (1 cup)

1 1/2 tablespoons chopped fresh or 1 1/2 teaspoons dried savory or basil leaves

1 clove garlic, finely chopped

1 can (15 to 16 ounces) black-eyed peas, rinsed and drained

1/2 cup shredded reduced-fat Monterey Jack cheese (2 ounces)

Heat broth, carrots, celery, onion, savory and garlic to boiling in 10-inch skillet; reduce heat to medium. Cook 8 to 10 minutes, stirring occasionally, until vegetables are tender. Stir in peas. Cook, stirring occasionally, until hot. Sprinkle with cheese.

1 Serving:		% Daily Value:	
Calories	160	Vitamin A	86%
Calories from fat	25	Vitamin C	8%
Fat, g	3	Calcium	16%
Saturated, g	2	Iron	16%
Cholesterol, mg	10	**Diet Exchanges:**	
Sodium, mg	440	2 starch/bread	
Carbohydrate, g	29		
Dietary Fiber, g	8		
Protein, g	12		

Confetti Beans and Rice

PREP: 8 min; COOK: 25 min

4 SERVINGS

1/2 cup uncooked regular long grain rice

1/4 cup chopped green bell pepper

1/2 cup water

1/4 teaspoon salt

1/8 teaspoon pepper

1 small zucchini, sliced (1 cup)

1 can (15 to 16 ounces) kidney beans, rinsed and drained

1 can (16 ounces) stewed tomatoes, undrained

Heat all ingredients to boiling in 2-quart saucepan; reduce heat to low. Cover and simmer 20 minutes, stirring occasionally.

1 Serving:		% Daily Value:	
Calories	185	Vitamin A	8%
Calories from fat	10	Vitamin C	22%
Fat, g	1	Calcium	6%
Saturated, g	0	Iron	20%
Cholesterol, mg	0	**Diet Exchanges:**	
Sodium, mg	650	2 starch/bread	
Carbohydrate, g	41	2 vegetable	
Dietary Fiber, g	6		
Protein, g	9		

Vegetable Sauté with Black Beans and Couscous

PREP: 10 min; COOK: 8 min

4 SERVINGS

1 teaspoon olive or vegetable oil

1 medium red onion, thinly sliced

1 large red bell pepper, cut crosswise in half and thinly sliced

1 medium fennel bulb, cut into fourths and thinly sliced

2 tablespoons chopped fresh or 2 teaspoons dried oregano leaves

1/4 teaspoon crushed red pepper

2 cans (15 ounces each) black beans, rinsed and drained

2 cups hot cooked couscous

Heat oil in 10-inch skillet over medium-high heat. Cook onion, bell pepper and fennel in oil 2 to 3 minutes, stirring occasionally, until crisp-tender. Stir in oregano, red pepper and beans; reduce heat to low. Simmer uncovered 5 minutes. Serve with couscous.

1 Serving:		% Daily Value:	
Calories	355	Vitamin A	16%
Calories from fat	25	Vitamin C	48%
Fat, g	3	Calcium	18%
Saturated, g	1	Iron	30%
Cholesterol, mg	0	**Diet Exchanges:**	
Sodium, mg	670	5 starch/bread	
Carbohydrate, g	78		
Dietary Fiber, g	17		
Protein, g	21		

Summer Lima Bean Soup

PREP: 8 min; COOK: 20 min

4 SERVINGS

A light, yet filling summer soup that's lovely either hot or cold; garnish with fat-free yogurt or sour cream.

2 cups frozen lima beans

1 cup frozen green peas

3 cups ready-to-serve fat-free reduced-sodium chicken broth

1/2 teaspoon salt

1/2 teaspoon dried thyme leaves

8 medium green onions, chopped (1/2 cup)

1 small bell pepper, diced (1/2 cup)

2 tablespoons pesto

Heat all ingredients except pesto to boiling in 2-quart saucepan; reduce heat to medium. Cook 15 minutes, stirring occasionally. Pour soup and pesto into blender or food processor. Cover and blend on high speed until smooth. Serve warm or cold.

1 Serving:		% Daily Value:	
Calories	150	Vitamin A	6%
Calories from fat	55	Vitamin C	22%
Fat, g	6	Calcium	6%
Saturated, g	1	Iron	12%
Cholesterol, mg	0	**Diet Exchanges:**	
Sodium, mg	720	1 starch/bread	
Carbohydrate, g	24	2 vegetable	
Dietary Fiber, g	9	1/2 fat	
Protein, g	9		

Italian Three-Bean Soup

PREP: 2 min; COOK: 30 min

4 SERVINGS

A simpler version of minestrone, this hearty soup uses canned beans and is seasoned with a touch of pesto.

2 cups frozen onion, bell pepper and green beans (from 16-ounce package)

1 3/4 cups ready-to-serve fat-free reduced-sodium chicken broth

1 teaspoon Italian seasoning

5 cloves garlic, finely chopped

1 can (16 ounces) stewed tomatoes, undrained

1 can (15 to 16 ounces) pinto beans, undrained

1 can (15 to 16 ounces) great northern beans, undrained

2 tablespoons pesto

Heat all ingredients except pesto to boiling in 3-quart saucepan; reduce heat to low. Cover and simmer 25 minutes, stirring occasionally. Stir in pesto.

1 Serving:		% Daily Value:	
Calories	255	Vitamin A	10%
Calories from fat	55	Vitamin C	18%
Fat, g	6	Calcium	18%
Saturated, g	1	Iron	30%
Cholesterol, mg	0	**Diet Exchanges:**	
Sodium, mg	740	3 starch/bread	
Carbohydrate, g	49	1 vegetable	
Dietary Fiber, g	14		
Protein, g	15		

Autumn Squash and Garbanzo Bean Soup

PREP: 5 min; COOK: 35 min

4 SERVINGS

Pureed garbanzo beans create a rich base for this hearty soup, and the squash colors the soup with the golden hue of autumn. If you'd like to save some time, cook the squash in the microwave.

1 can (15 to 16 ounces) garbanzo beans, rinsed and drained

3 cups ready-to-serve fat-free reduced-sodium chicken broth

2 cups mashed cooked buttercup or acorn squash

1 medium onion, chopped (1/2 cup)

1 teaspoon ground cumin

1/2 teaspoon ground coriander

1 teaspoon salt

1/4 cup chopped fresh parsley

Place beans, broth and squash in blender or food processor. Cover and blend on high speed until smooth. Pour into 3-quart saucepan. Stir in remaining ingredients except parsley. Heat to boiling; reduce heat to low. Cover and simmer 30 minutes, stirring occasionally. Stir in parsley.

1 Serving:		% Daily Value:	
Calories	165	Vitamin A	44%
Calories from fat	25	Vitamin C	16%
Fat, g	3	Calcium	6%
Saturated, g	0	Iron	18%
Cholesterol, mg	0	**Diet Exchanges:**	
Sodium, mg	1090	2 starch/bread	
Carbohydrate, g	34	1 vegetable	
Dietary Fiber, g	8		
Protein, g	9		

METABOLISM

What is metabolism?

- It's the process of building up new substances that become part of our body structure or will be used to help our bodies function.

- It's the breaking down of certain materials into smaller units.

- It occurs in our cells.

What is metabolic rate?

- Metabolic rate is the rate of energy use in our bodies.

So what does this have to do with eating and exercise?

- We can help our metabolism along by balancing our food intake with energy-burning exercise.

Curried Lentil and Barley Casserole

PREP: 5 min; COOK: 49 min

4 SERVINGS

Curry lovers may want to add another 1/2 to 1 teaspoon curry powder to this hearty dish.

1/4 cup dried lentils, sorted and rinsed

2 cups ready-to-serve fat-free reduced-sodium chicken broth

1 teaspoon curry powder

3 cloves garlic, finely chopped

3/4 cup uncooked quick-cooking barley

1 package (16 ounces) frozen corn, green peas and carrots

4 ounces feta cheese, crumbled

Heat lentils, broth, curry powder and garlic to boiling in 3-quart saucepan; reduce heat to low. Cover and simmer 30 minutes, stirring occasionally.

Stir in barley and vegetables. Heat to boiling; reduce heat to low. Cover and simmer 10 to 15 minutes, stirring occasionally, until lentils and barley are tender and liquid is absorbed. Sprinkle with cheese.

1 Serving:		% Daily Value:	
Calories	305	Vitamin A	62%
Calories from fat	70	Vitamin C	4%
Fat, g	8	Calcium	20%
Saturated, g	5	Iron	20%
Cholesterol, mg	25	**Diet Exchanges:**	
Sodium, mg	760	3 starch/bread	
Carbohydrate, g	67	2 vegetable	
Dietary Fiber, g	16		
Protein, g	17		

Cuban Spicy Bean Salad with Oranges and Cilantro

PREP: 10 min; STAND: 30 min

4 SERVINGS

A sweet and spicy dressing highlights the flavor of oranges and cilantro in this Caribbean salad.

2 oranges, peeled and sliced, or 1 can (11 ounces) mandarin orange segments in light syrup, drained

2 cups shredded carrots (3 medium)

2/3 cup chopped fresh cilantro

1/2 cup balsamic or red wine vinegar

2 tablespoons sugar

2 teaspoons chopped fresh or canned jalapeño chilies

2 cans (15 ounces each) black beans, rinsed and drained

4 cups bite-size pieces curly endive or lettuce

Mix all ingredients except endive in nonmetal bowl. Cover and let stand 30 minutes. Divide endive among 4 salad plates. Top with bean mixture.

1 Serving:		% Daily Value:	
Calories	310	Vitamin A	100%
Calories from fat	20	Vitamin C	48%
Fat, g	2	Calcium	20%
Saturated, g	0	Iron	32%
Cholesterol, mg	0	**Diet Exchanges:**	
Sodium, mg	460	2 starch/bread	
Carbohydrate, g	74	1 vegetable	
Dietary Fiber, g	18		
Protein, g	18		

Cuban Spicy Bean Salad with Oranges and Cilantro

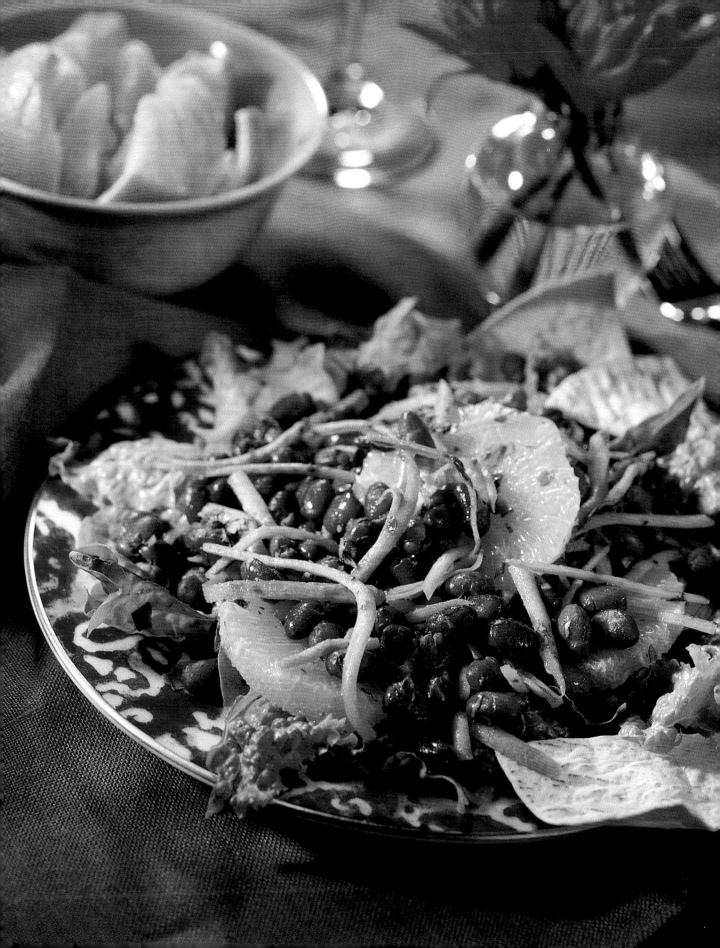

Moroccan Bulgur

PREP: 6 min; COOK: 15 min; STAND: 20 min

4 SERVINGS

Bulgur, also called cracked wheat, is a fast-cooking staple of Middle Eastern cuisines.

3 cups sliced mushrooms (8 ounces)

2 large onions, chopped (2 cups)

2 cloves garlic, finely chopped

3 cups frozen green peas, red bell pepper and broccoli (from 16-ounce package)

1 1/2 cups uncooked bulgur

1/4 cup currants or raisins

2 teaspoons curry powder

1/2 teaspoon salt

2 cups boiling water

Spray 10-inch nonstick skillet with nonstick cooking spray; heat over medium-high heat. Cook mushrooms, onions and garlic in skillet about 8 minutes, stirring occasionally, until onions are tender.

Stir in remaining ingredients except water. Cook 2 minutes, stirring occasionally. Stir in water. Heat to boiling; remove from heat. Cover and let stand 15 to 20 minutes or until water is absorbed.

1 Serving:		% Daily Value:	
Calories	245	Vitamin A	36%
Calories from fat	10	Vitamin C	36%
Fat, g	1	Calcium	8%
Saturated, g	0	Iron	18%
Cholesterol, mg	0	**Diet Exchanges:**	
Sodium, mg	340	4 starch/bread	
Carbohydrate, g	63		
Dietary Fiber, g	15		
Protein, g	11		

Polenta with Cheese

PREP: 5 min; COOK: 20 min; BAKE: 20 min

4 SERVINGS

1 cup yellow cornmeal

3/4 cup water

3 1/4 cups boiling water

2 teaspoons salt

1 tablespoon reduced-calorie spread

1 cup grated fat-free Parmesan cheese

1/3 cup shredded reduced-fat Swiss cheese

Heat oven to 350°. Grease 1 1/2-quart casserole. Mix cornmeal and 3/4 cup water in 2-quart saucepan. Stir in boiling water and salt. Cook, stirring constantly, until mixture thickens and boils; reduce heat to low. Cover and simmer 10 minutes, stirring occasionally; remove from heat. Stir until smooth.

Spread one-third of the cornmeal mixture in casserole. Dot with 1 teaspoon of the spread. Sprinkle with 1/3 cup of the Parmesan cheese. Repeat layers twice with remaining cornmeal mixture, spread and Parmesan cheese. Sprinkle with Swiss cheese. Bake uncovered 15 to 20 minutes or until hot.

1 Serving:		% Daily Value:	
Calories	250	Vitamin A	12%
Calories from fat	25	Vitamin C	0%
Fat, g	3	Calcium	34%
Saturated, g	1	Iron	8%
Cholesterol, mg	5	**Diet Exchanges:**	
Sodium, mg	1610	2 starch/bread	
Carbohydrate, g	41	1 skim milk	
Dietary Fiber, g	2		
Protein, g	17		

Polenta with Cheese

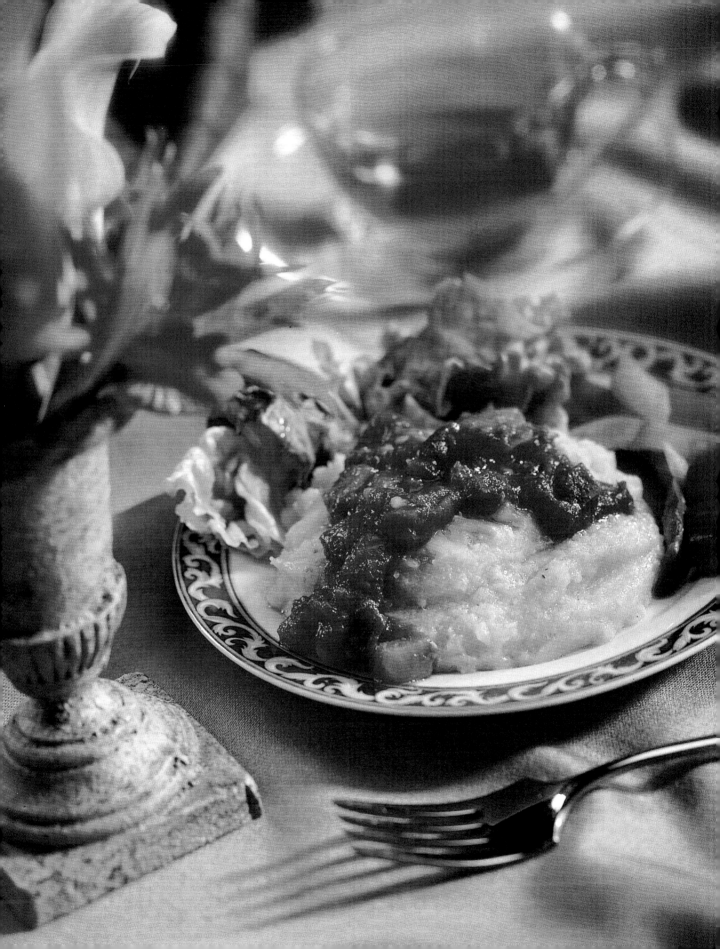

Sweet Potato Polenta

PREP: 5 min; COOK: 7 min; BAKE: 45 min

4 SERVINGS

Mashed cooked sweet potatoes lend a beautiful golden color to this easy Italian dish. To speed preparation, cook sweet potatoes in your microwave oven following manufacturer's directions.

**4 medium sweet potatoes or yams
   (2 pounds)**

**2 1/2 cups ready-to-serve fat-free reduced-
   sodium chicken broth**

2 teaspoons reduced-sodium soy sauce

1/2 teaspoon ground nutmeg

1 3/4 cups yellow cornmeal

2 cloves garlic, finely chopped

**1/4 cup shredded reduced-fat mozzarella
   cheese (1 ounce)**

Heat oven to 375°. Pierce each potato several times with fork. Bake about 45 minutes or until tender; cool. Peel and mash sweet potatoes.

Mix 1 1/2 cups of the broth, the soy sauce, nutmeg and cornmeal in medium bowl. Heat remaining 1 cup broth and the garlic to boiling in 3-quart saucepan. Stir in cornmeal mixture; reduce heat to medium. Cook about 5 minutes, stirring frequently, until liquid is absorbed. Stir in mashed sweet potatoes; cook until hot. Sprinkle with cheese.

1 Serving:		% Daily Value:	
Calories	330	Vitamin A	100%
Calories from fat	20	Vitamin C	24%
Fat, g	2	Calcium	8%
Saturated, g	1	Iron	18%
Cholesterol, mg	0	**Diet Exchanges:**	
Sodium, mg	430	5 starch/bread	
Carbohydrate, g	77		
Dietary Fiber, g	8		
Protein, g	9		

Spicy Couscous with Chilie and Vegetables

PREP: 8 min; COOK: 7 min; STAND: 10 min

4 SERVINGS

**2 1/4 cups ready-to-serve fat-free reduced-
   sodium chicken broth**

**1 package (16 ounces) frozen corn, broccoli
   and sweet red peppers**

1 cup uncooked couscous

**2 teaspoons chopped fresh or canned
   jalapeño chilies**

3 tablespoons reduced-sodium soy sauce

2 teaspoons sesame or vegetable oil

1 tablespoon honey or packed brown sugar

1/4 cup chopped fresh cilantro

Heat broth to boiling in 3-quart saucepan. Stir in vegetable mixture. Heat 1 minute; remove vegetables with slotted spoon. Set aside and keep warm. Heat broth to boiling again. Stir in couscous and chilies; remove from heat. Cover and let stand 10 minutes.

Beat soy sauce, oil, honey and cilantro in medium bowl, using wire whisk. Add vegetables; toss. Spoon couscous on serving platter. Top with vegetable mixture.

1 Serving:		% Daily Value:	
Calories	235	Vitamin A	36%
Calories from fat	25	Vitamin C	30%
Fat, g	3	Calcium	6%
Saturated, g	0	Iron	8%
Cholesterol, mg	0	**Diet Exchanges:**	
Sodium, mg	740	2 starch/bread	
Carbohydrate, g	47	3 vegetable	
Dietary Fiber, g	5		
Protein, g	10		

Spicy Couscous with Chilies and Vegetables

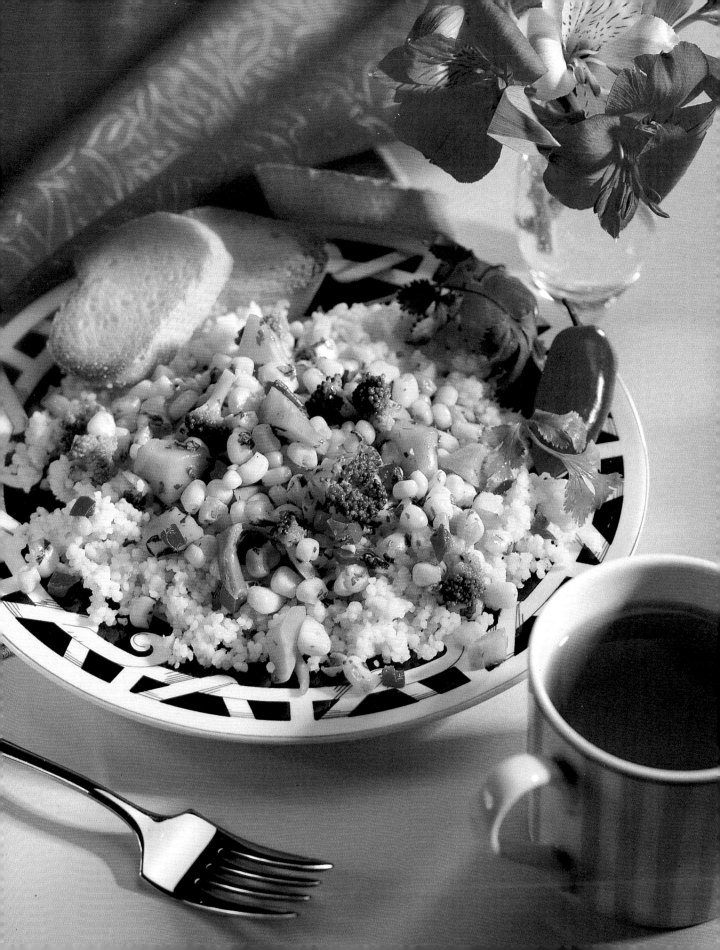

Couscous Timbales

PREP: 5 min; COOK: 4 min; STAND: 5 min; BAKE: 20 min

5 SERVINGS

Timbales are molded grain dishes that are easy to make in small custard cups or ramekins and elegant to serve. Garnish them with low-fat yogurt and chopped fresh parsley.

3 medium green onions, sliced (1/3 cup)

3/4 teaspoon ground cumin

1/4 teaspoon salt

1/4 teaspoon ground turmeric

1/4 teaspoon ground cinnamon

1 can (16 ounces) whole tomatoes, drained and chopped

1/4 cup currants or raisins

1 cup water

3/4 cup uncooked couscous

Heat oven to 400°. Spray 2-quart saucepan with nonstick cooking spray; heat over medium-high heat. Cook onions in skillet 1 minute, stirring frequently. Stir in cumin, salt, turmeric, cinnamon, tomatoes, currants and water. Heat to boiling. Stir in couscous; remove from heat. Cover and let stand 5 minutes.

Spray five 6-ounce custard cups or ramekins with nonstick cooking spray. Spoon couscous mixture into custard cups; press down lightly. Place custard cups on cookie sheet. Bake about 20 minutes or until set. Carefully run knife around edge of custard cups to loosen timbales; invert timbales onto individual serving plates.

1 Serving:		% Daily Value:	
Calories	140	Vitamin A	6%
Calories from fat	8	Vitamin C	12%
Fat, g	1	Calcium	4%
Saturated, g	0	Iron	8%
Cholesterol, mg	0	**Diet Exchanges:**	
Sodium, mg	232	2 starch/bread	
Carbohydrate, g	30	1 vegetable	
Dietary Fiber, g	3		
Protein, g	5		

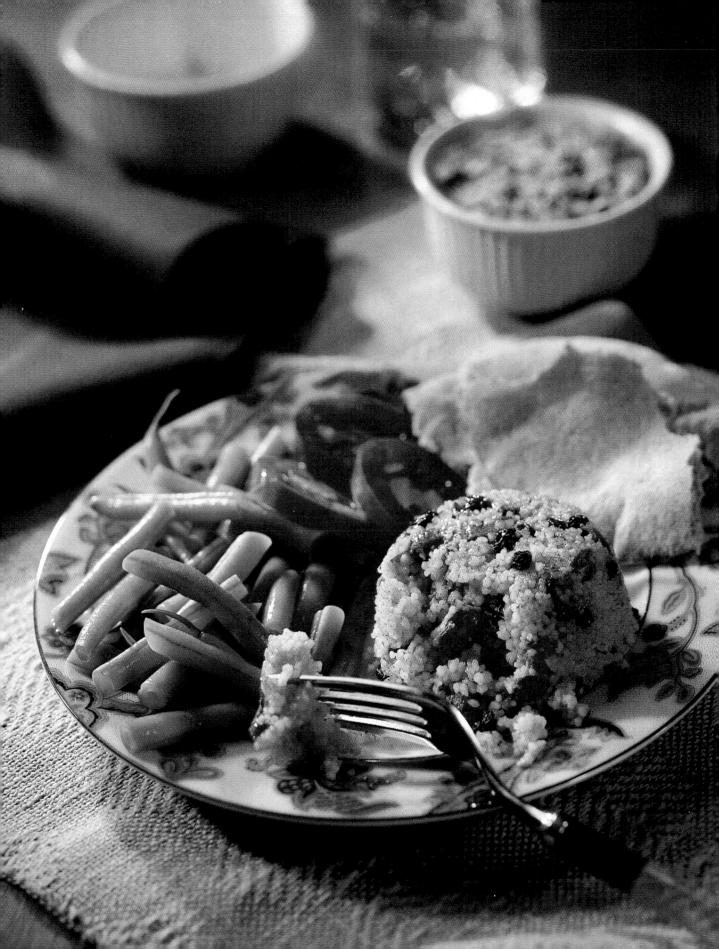

Spinach Orzo

PREP: 8 min; COOK: 23 min

4 SERVINGS

2 teaspoons reduced-calorie spread

2 cloves garlic, finely chopped

1 small carrot, shredded (1/2 cup)

4 cups ready-to-serve fat-free reduced-sodium chicken broth

2 cups uncooked rosamarina (orzo) pasta

1 package (10 ounces) frozen chopped spinach, thawed and squeezed to drain

1/2 cup grated fat-free Parmesan cheese

1 teaspoon dried basil leaves

Melt spread in 3-quart saucepan over medium heat. Cook garlic and carrot in spread about 2 minutes, stirring occasionally, until carrot is tender. Stir in broth, pasta and spinach. Heat to boiling; reduce heat to low. Cover and simmer 15 to 20 minutes or until broth is absorbed. Stir in cheese and basil before serving.

1 Serving:		% Daily Value:	
Calories	310	Vitamin A	60%
Calories from fat	40	Vitamin C	4%
Fat, g	4	Calcium	24%
Saturated, g	2	Iron	20%
Cholesterol, mg	10	**Diet Exchanges:**	
Sodium, mg	680	2 starch/bread	
Carbohydrate, g	56	4 vegetable	
Dietary Fiber, g	4		
Protein, g	16		

Savory Millet and Potato Stew

PREP: 8 min; COOK: 25 min

4 SERVINGS

Thick and rich, this polenta-like stew is made with millet, a high-protein, low-fat grain.

5 cups ready-to-serve fat-free reduced-sodium chicken broth

2 tablespoons reduced-sodium soy sauce

1 package (16 ounces) frozen carrots, cauliflower and red bell pepper

1 cup diced red potatoes

1 cup uncooked millet

1 teaspoon dried thyme leaves

1/4 to 1/2 teaspoon pepper

1 large onion, chopped (1 cup)

4 cloves garlic, finely chopped

Heat broth and soy sauce to boiling in 4-quart saucepan. Stir in remaining ingredients. Heat to boiling; reduce heat to medium. Cover and cook 12 to 16 minutes, stirring occasionally, until millet and potatoes are tender.

1 Serving:		% Daily Value:	
Calories	255	Vitamin A	36%
Calories from fat	25	Vitamin C	36%
Fat, g	3	Calcium	6%
Saturated, g	1	Iron	14%
Cholesterol, mg	0	**Diet Exchanges:**	
Sodium, mg	720	3 starch/bread	
Carbohydrate, g	54	2 vegetable	
Dietary Fiber, g	8		
Protein, g	11		

Savory Southwest Loaf

PREP: 5 min; BAKE: 35 min; STAND: 10 min

6 SERVINGS

Serve this loaf with a zesty salsa and chopped fresh cilantro.

2 3/4 cups cooked bulgur

1 cup cooked brown or white rice

1 cup fat-free sour cream

3/4 cup shredded reduced-fat Monterey Jack cheese (3 ounces)

1 teaspoon chili powder

2 cans (4 ounces each) chopped green chilies, undrained

Heat oven to 350°. Mix all ingredients in ungreased loaf pan, 9 × 5 × 3 inches. Bake uncovered 30 to 35 minutes or until set. Let stand 10 minutes before slicing.

1 Serving:		% Daily Value:	
Calories	165	Vitamin A	12%
Calories from fat	25	Vitamin C	22%
Fat, g	3	Calcium	20%
Saturated, g	2	Iron	4%
Cholesterol, mg	10	**Diet Exchanges:**	
Sodium, mg	570	2 starch/bread	
Carbohydrate, g	30		
Dietary Fiber, g	5		
Protein, g	10		

FANTASTIC, IT'S FAT FREE! BUT BEWARE . . .

Advice about dieting is everywhere—much of it is factual and reasonable, much of it is not. Since our nation has embraced the low-fat/no-fat mantra, many diets have promoted the idea of only watching fat intake to achieve weight loss. Then a funny thing happened. People didn't lose weight, they gained weight! Why? The reason is simple: Too many calories were consumed because calories were not taken into consideration. Calories are calories, whether they come from chocolate fudge cake or fat-free chocolate cookies. Although losing weight isn't always easy, the formula for losing it is:

Calories Consumed vs. Calories Burned

More calories must be burned than consumed in order to lose weight. Fat-free foods certainly can help significantly in a weight loss plan, but they can also offer a false sense of diet security. Just because foods are fat-free doesn't mean they are low-calorie too. For example, just one small fat-free fruit-filled cookie contains fifty calories. Many people overeat fat-free foods believing there are no consequences. It's easy to eat half of a box of fat-free cookies or a pint of fat-free ice cream in a day's time. Indeed they have no fat, but your daily calorie intake will soar unless you are aware of and count your calories. Check out our handy Calorie Chart on pages 247–252 to help keep on track.

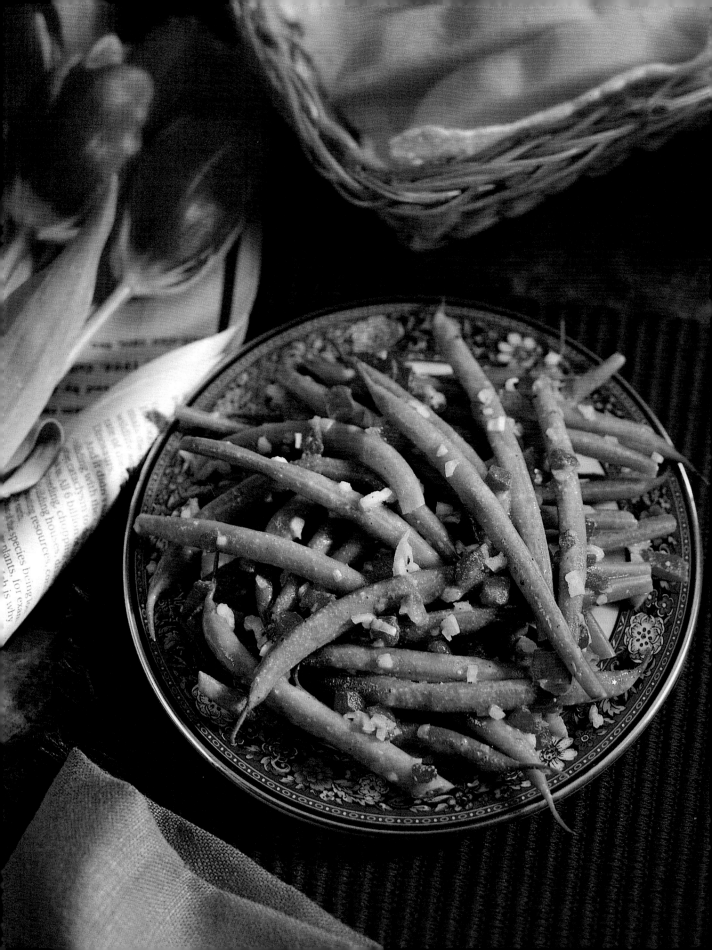

9

Savory Breads, Vegetables and Side Dishes

Green Beans with Pimento Sauce
(page 205)

Popovers

PREP: 8 min; BAKE: 40 min

6 POPOVERS

1 egg

2 egg whites

1 cup all-purpose flour

1 cup skim milk

1/4 teaspoon salt

Heat oven to 450°. Spray six 6-ounce custard cups with nonstick cooking spray. Place all ingredients in blender in order listed. Cover and blend on medium speed about 15 seconds, stopping blender to scrape sides if necessary, just until smooth. Fill custard cups about half full. Bake 20 minutes.

Reduce oven temperature to 350°. Bake 15 to 20 minutes longer or until deep golden brown. Immediately remove from cups. Serve hot.

1 Popover:		% Daily Value:	
Calories	105	Vitamin A	4%
Calories from fat	10	Vitamin C	0%
Fat, g	1	Calcium	6%
Saturated, g	0	Iron	6%
Cholesterol, mg	35	**Diet Exchanges:**	
Sodium, mg	150	1 starch/bread	
Carbohydrate, g	18	1/2 skim milk	
Dietary Fiber, g	0		
Protein, g	6		

Chewy Pizza Bread

PREP: 10 min; BAKE: 20 min

6 SERVINGS

The taste of pizza without all the fat!

1 1/2 cups all-purpose flour

1 1/2 teaspoons baking powder

1/2 teaspoon salt

3/4 cup regular or nonalcoholic beer

1/2 cup spaghetti sauce

1/3 cup shredded reduced-fat mozzarella cheese

Chopped fresh basil leaves, if desired

Heat oven to 425°. Spray round pan, 9 × 1 1/2 inches, with nonstick cooking spray. Mix flour, baking powder and salt in medium bowl. Stir in beer just until flour is moistened.

Spread dough in pan. Spread spaghetti sauce over dough. Sprinkle with cheese. Bake 15 to 20 minutes or until toothpick inserted in center comes out clean. Sprinkle with basil. Serve warm.

1 Serving:		% Daily Value:	
Calories	145	Vitamin A	4%
Calories from fat	20	Vitamin C	0%
Fat, g	2	Calcium	12%
Saturated, g	0	Iron	10%
Cholesterol, mg	0	**Diet Exchanges:**	
Sodium, mg	500	2 starch/bread	
Carbohydrate, g	29		
Dietary Fiber, g	1		
Protein, g	4		

Dill Casserole Bread

PREP: 10 min; BAKE: 35 min

8 SERVINGS

Change the flavor of this quick bread by substituting dried basil for the dill weed.

1 cup skim milk

2 tablespoons reduced-calorie spread, melted

1 egg white

2 1/4 cups Bisquick Reduced Fat baking mix

3 tablespoons finely chopped onion

1 1/4 teaspoons dried dill weed

Heat oven to 375°. Spray 1-quart round casserole with nonstick cooking spray. Beat milk, spread and egg white in medium bowl until smooth. Stir in remaining ingredients just until baking mix is moistened (batter will be lumpy). Spread batter in casserole.

Bake about 35 minutes or until toothpick inserted in center comes out clean. Cool 5 minutes; remove from casserole. Serve warm.

1 Serving:		% Daily Value:	
Calories	145	Vitamin A	6%
Calories from fat	35	Vitamin C	0%
Fat, g	4	Calcium	6%
Saturated, g	1	Iron	6%
Cholesterol, mg	0	**Diet Exchanges:**	
Sodium, mg	430	1 1/2 starch/bread	
Carbohydrate, g	24	1/2 fat	
Dietary Fiber, g	1		
Protein, g	4		

Tomato-Basil Biscuits

PREP: 15 min; BAKE: 10 min

8 SERVINGS

Sun-dried tomatoes add a slightly chewy texture to these biscuits.

8 sun-dried tomato halves (not oil-packed)

1 1/2 cups all-purpose flour

1 1/2 teaspoons baking powder

1/4 teaspoon baking soda

1/2 teaspoon salt

1 tablespoon chopped fresh or 1 teaspoon dried basil leaves

3/4 cup low-fat buttermilk

3 tablespoons vegetable oil

Heat oven to 450°. Pour enough hot water over sun-dried tomatoes to cover. Let stand 10 to 15 minutes or until softened; drain and chop.

Mix flour, baking powder, baking soda, salt, basil and tomatoes in medium bowl. Mix buttermilk and oil; stir into flour mixture until soft dough forms. Drop dough by 8 spoonfuls onto ungreased cookie sheet. Bake 8 to 10 minutes or until golden brown. Serve warm.

1 Serving:		% Daily Value:	
Calories	140	Vitamin A	0%
Calories from fat	55	Vitamin C	0%
Fat, g	6	Calcium	8%
Saturated, g	1	Iron	8%
Cholesterol, mg	0	**Diet Exchanges:**	
Sodium, mg	340	1 starch/bread	
Carbohydrate, g	20	1 vegetable	
Dietary Fiber, g	1	1 fat	
Protein, g	3		

Irish Yogurt Bread

PREP: 10 min; BAKE: 25 min

8 SERVINGS

1 3/4 cups all-purpose flour

1/2 cup currants or raisins

1 1/2 teaspoons baking powder

1/4 teaspoon baking soda

1/4 teaspoon salt

1 container (8 ounces) lemon, orange or
    plain low-fat yogurt

2 tablespoons vegetable oil

Heat oven to 375°. Spray round pan, 9 × 1 1/2 inches, with nonstick cooking spray. Mix flour, currants, baking powder, baking soda and salt in medium bowl. Mix yogurt and oil; stir into flour mixture just until flour is moistened.

Spread dough in pan. Bake 20 to 25 minutes or until toothpick inserted in center comes out clean. Serve warm or cool.

1 Serving:		% Daily Value:	
Calories	170	Vitamin A	0%
Calories from fat	35	Vitamin C	0%
Fat, g	4	Calcium	10%
Saturated, g	1	Iron	8%
Cholesterol, mg	2	**Diet Exchanges:**	
Sodium, mg	220	2 starch/bread	
Carbohydrate, g	30		
Dietary Fiber, g	1		
Protein, g	4		

Carrot-Zucchini Muffins

PREP: 15 min; BAKE: 25 min

12 MUFFINS

Kids will like these muffins with a glass of milk for an after-school snack.

2/3 cup skim milk

1/4 cup fat-free cholesterol-free egg product
    or 2 egg whites

2 tablespoons vegetable oil

2 cups Bisquick Reduced Fat baking mix

2 tablespoons sugar

1 teaspoon grated lemon peel

1 small carrot, shredded (1/2 cup)

1/2 cup shredded zucchini

Heat oven to 400°. Spray 12 medium muffin cups, 2 1/2 × 1 1/4 inches, with nonstick cooking spray, or line with paper baking cups. Beat milk, egg product and oil in large bowl until smooth. Stir in baking mix, sugar and lemon peel just until baking mix is moistened (batter will be lumpy). Fold in carrot and zucchini.

Fill cups about three-fourths full. Bake 20 to 25 minutes or until golden brown. Immediately remove from pan. Cool on wire rack. Serve warm or cool.

1 Muffin:		% Daily Value:	
Calories	110	Vitamin A	8%
Calories from fat	35	Vitamin C	0%
Fat, g	4	Calcium	4%
Saturated, g	1	Iron	4%
Cholesterol, mg	0	**Diet Exchanges:**	
Sodium, mg	230	1 starch/bread	
Carbohydrate, g	17	1 fat	
Dietary Fiber, g	0		
Protein, g	2		

Irish Yogurt Bread, Carrot-Zucchini Muffins

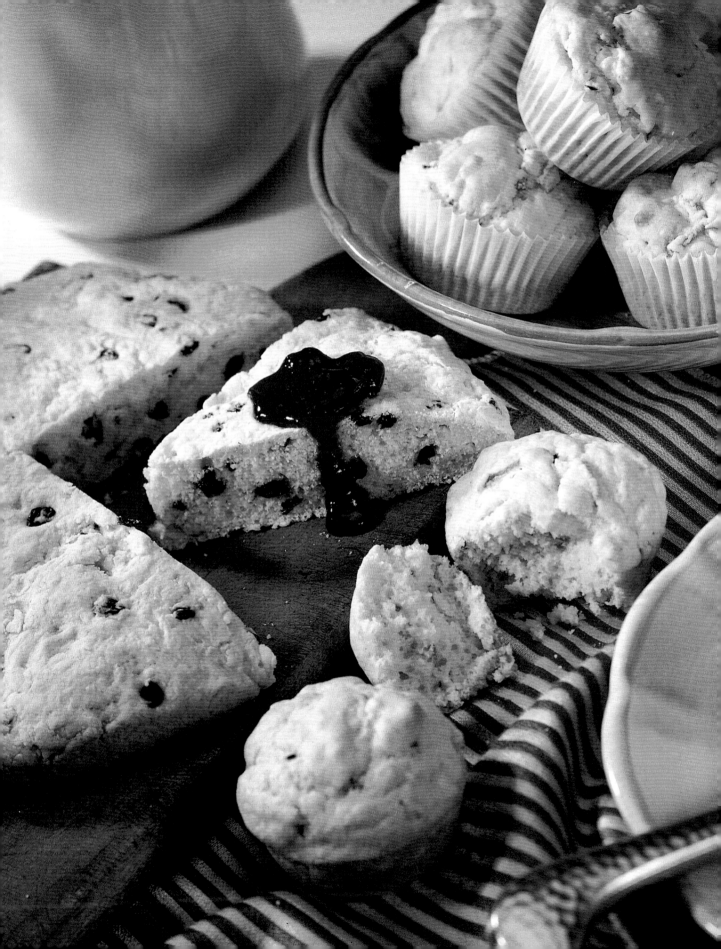

Maple-Ginger Squash

PREP: 10 min; BAKE: 45 min

4 SERVINGS

To make the squash easier and safer to cut, first microwave the whole, uncut squash on High power (100%) for 3 to 4 minutes, making quarter turns every minute or until slightly softened.

1 large acorn squash (2 pounds)

1/4 teaspoon salt

2 tablespoons maple-flavored syrup

2 teaspoons reduced-calorie spread, melted

1 teaspoon finely chopped gingerroot or 1/4 teaspoon ground ginger

Heat oven to 400°. Cut squash lengthwise into fourths; remove seeds and fibers. Place squash, cut sides up, in ungreased rectangular baking dish, 13 × 9 × 2 inches. Sprinkle with salt. Mix remaining ingredients; drizzle over squash. Bake uncovered about 45 minutes or until tender.

1 Serving:		% Daily Value:	
Calories	130	Vitamin A	10%
Calories from fat	10	Vitamin C	14%
Fat, g	1	Calcium	8%
Saturated, g	0	Iron	8%
Cholesterol, mg	0	**Diet Exchanges:**	
Sodium, mg	190	2 starch/bread	
Carbohydrate, g	33		
Dietary Fiber, g	5		
Protein, g	2		

Sweet Potatoes with Onion Topping

PREP: 10 min; COOK: 6 min; BAKE: 45 min

4 SERVINGS

Caramelized onions add a special sweet-sour flavor to baked sweet potatoes.

4 medium sweet potatoes (1 1/2 pounds)

1 tablespoon reduced-calorie spread

1 large onion, chopped (1 cup)

1 tablespoon packed brown sugar

1 tablespoon balsamic or red wine vinegar

Heat oven to 375°. Pierce each potato several times with fork. Bake about 45 minutes or until tender.

While sweet potatoes are baking, melt spread in 8-inch skillet over medium heat. Cook onion in spread about 5 minutes, stirring occasionally, until tender. Stir in brown sugar and vinegar; cover and remove from heat. Make lengthwise cut in each sweet potato. Top with onion mixture.

1 Serving:		% Daily Value:	
Calories	145	Vitamin A	100%
Calories from fat	20	Vitamin C	24%
Fat, g	2	Calcium	4%
Saturated, g	0	Iron	4%
Cholesterol, mg	0	**Diet Exchanges:**	
Sodium, mg	50	2 starch/bread	
Carbohydrate, g	34	1 vegetable	
Dietary Fiber, g	4		
Protein, g	2		

Green Beans with Pimiento Sauce

PREP: 10 min; COOK: 12 min

4 SERVINGS

Steaming is an excellent way to preserve the vitamin content of vegetables—you can also microwave vegetables for excellent results.

1 pound green beans

1 jar (2 ounces) diced pimientos, drained

2 tablespoons finely chopped shallot or onion

1 tablespoon white wine vinegar

1 1/2 teaspoons Dijon mustard

1/8 teaspoon pepper

Place steamer basket in 1/2 inch water in saucepan or skillet (water should not touch bottom of basket). Place green beans in basket. Cover tightly and heat to boiling; reduce heat to low. Steam 10 to 12 minutes or until crisp-tender; drain.

While beans are steaming, mix remaining ingredients. Toss beans and pimiento sauce. Serve immediately.

1 Serving:

Calories	30	**% Daily Value:**	
Calories from fat	0	Vitamin A	8%
Fat, g	0	Vitamin C	14%
Saturated, g	0	Calcium	4%
Cholesterol, mg	0	Iron	6%
Sodium, mg	35	**Diet Exchanges:**	
Carbohydrate, g	8	1 vegetable	
Dietary Fiber, g	3		
Protein, g	2		

Asparagus with Tomatoes

PREP: 10 min; COOK: 21 min

4 SERVINGS

Asparagus is best served crisp-tender, so be careful not to overcook it.

2 teaspoons vegetable oil

1 small onion, chopped (1/4 cup)

3 roma (plum) tomatoes, chopped

1 tablespoon lemon juice

1 tablespoon honey

1/4 teaspoon salt

1 1/2 pounds asparagus

Heat oil in 10-inch skillet over medium heat. Cook onion in oil 2 to 3 minutes, stirring occasionally, until tender. Stir in tomatoes, lemon juice, honey and salt. Cook 1 minute, stirring occasionally. Remove mixture from skillet; keep warm.

Wipe out skillet. Heat 1 inch water to boiling in skillet. Add asparagus. Heat to boiling; reduce heat to medium. Cook covered 10 to 17 minutes or until stalk ends are crisp-tender; drain. Place asparagus in serving dish. Top with tomato mixture.

1 Serving:

Calories	85	**% Daily Value:**	
Calories from fat	25	Vitamin A	10%
Fat, g	3	Vitamin C	28%
Saturated, g	1	Calcium	2%
Cholesterol, mg	0	Iron	4%
Sodium, mg	160	**Diet Exchanges:**	
Carbohydrate, g	13	1 starch/bread	
Dietary Fiber, g	2		
Protein, g	3		

Honey-Mint Carrots

PREP: 10 min; COOK: 12 min

6 SERVINGS

**3 cups 1/4-inch diagonal slices carrots*
(about 6 medium)**

1 tablespoon honey

**1 tablespoon chopped fresh or 1 teaspoon
dried mint leaves**

Heat 1 inch water to boiling in 2-quart saucepan.
Add carrots. Heat to boiling; reduce heat to low.
Cover and simmer about 10 minutes or until crisp-
tender; drain. Toss with honey and mint.

**1 package (16 ounces) frozen sliced carrots, cooked and
drained, can be substituted for the cooked fresh carrots.*

1 Serving:		% Daily Value:	
Calories	35	Vitamin A	100%
Calories from fat	0	Vitamin C	4%
Fat, g	0	Calcium	2%
Saturated, g	0	Iron	2%
Cholesterol, mg	0	**Diet Exchanges:**	
Sodium, mg	25	2 vegetable	
Carbohydrate, g	10		
Dietary Fiber, g	2		
Protein, g	1		

Gingered Spinach

PREP: 10 min; COOK: 5 min

4 SERVINGS

*If you'd like to save on preparation time, purchase
prewashed spinach.*

1 teaspoon vegetable oil

1/4 teaspoon sesame oil

1/2 pound spinach

2 teaspoons finely chopped gingerroot

1 teaspoon reduced-sodium soy sauce

1 cup julienne strips jicama (4 ounces)

2 teaspoons sesame seed, toasted

Heat vegetable and sesame oils in 10-inch nonstick
skillet over medium-high heat. Cook half of the
spinach, the gingerroot and soy sauce in oils, stirring occasionally, until spinach begins to wilt.

Stir in remaining spinach and the jicama. Cook
about 2 minutes, stirring frequently, until spinach is
wilted and jicama is hot. Sprinkle with sesame seed.

1 Serving:		% Daily Value:	
Calories	35	Vitamin A	34%
Calories from fat	20	Vitamin C	14%
Fat, g	2	Calcium	4%
Saturated, g	0	Iron	8%
Cholesterol, mg	0	**Diet Exchanges:**	
Sodium, mg	85	1 vegetable	
Carbohydrate, g	5		
Dietary Fiber, g	3		
Protein, g	2		

Southwest Pepper Skillet

PREP: 12 min; COOK: 5 min

6 SERVINGS

Choose different colors of peppers for this pretty dish.

1 teaspoon olive or vegetable oil

4 small bell peppers, cut into strips

1 medium onion, thinly sliced

2 cloves garlic, finely chopped

1 tablespoon chopped fresh cilantro

1 teaspoon cumin seed

Heat oil in 10-inch nonstick skillet over medium-high heat. Cook remaining ingredients in oil 4 to 5 minutes, stirring occasionally, until peppers are crisp-tender.

1 Serving:		% Daily Value:	
Calories	25	Vitamin A	2%
Calories from fat	10	Vitamin C	24%
Fat, g	1	Calcium	0%
Saturated, g	0	Iron	2%
Cholesterol, mg	0	**Diet Exchanges:**	
Sodium, mg	0	1 vegetable	
Carbohydrate, g	4		
Dietary Fiber, g	1		
Protein, g	1		

SKINNY GARLIC BREAD

Have you ever eaten garlic bread that just oozes with fat? In fact, so much fat that it could literally be squeezed out? If you still crave that buttery, cheesy taste but want less fat, try one of these easy and clever techniques.

Lower-fat garlic bread can be made by using partially or completely frozen slices of French, Italian or baguette bread. Because the surface of frozen bread is hard and not spongy or porous, it can be spread with a very thin and even layer of margarine, butter or spread. Or, if you prefer, spray fresh bread slices with butter- or olive oil–flavored nonstick cooking spray. Sprinkle bread with garlic powder and fat-free Parmesan cheese.

Another great way to serve bread is to toast the slices first and then top them with chopped fresh tomatoes, garlic and fresh basil or chopped bell peppers, green onion and capers, to name a few. *Bon appétit!*

Festive Broccoli and Corn

PREP: 8 min; COOK: 10 min

4 SERVINGS

1 package (10 ounces) frozen broccoli cuts or broccoli flowerets

1 cup frozen whole kernel corn

1 medium onion, chopped (1/2 cup)

1/2 cup water

2 teaspoons chopped fresh or 1/2 teaspoon dried basil leaves

1/2 teaspoon chicken bouillon granules

1 clove garlic, finely chopped

1 jar (2 ounces) diced pimientos, drained

Heat all ingredients to boiling in 1-quart saucepan; reduce heat to low. Cover and simmer 4 to 5 minutes or until broccoli is crisp-tender.

1 Serving:		% Daily Value:	
Calories	55	Vitamin A	16%
Calories from fat	0	Vitamin C	32%
Fat, g	0	Calcium	4%
Saturated, g	0	Iron	4%
Cholesterol, mg	0	**Diet Exchanges:**	
Sodium, mg	180	2 vegetable	
Carbohydrate, g	14		
Dietary Fiber, g	3		
Protein, g	3		

Vegetable Confetti

PREP: 10 min

4 SERVINGS

A quick, colorful salad that can be made a day in advance.

2 medium carrots, shredded (1 1/2 cups)

1 small zucchini, shredded (1 cup)

1 medium bell pepper, chopped (1 cup)

1/4 cup fat-free Italian dressing

1/4 teaspoon pepper

Mix all ingredients in nonmetal bowl.

1 Serving:		% Daily Value:	
Calories	30	Vitamin A	58%
Calories from fat	0	Vitamin C	40%
Fat, g	0	Calcium	2%
Saturated, g	0	Iron	2%
Cholesterol, mg	0	**Diet Exchanges:**	
Sodium, mg	130	1 vegetable	
Carbohydrate, g	8		
Dietary Fiber, g	2		
Protein, g	1		

Vegetable Confetti

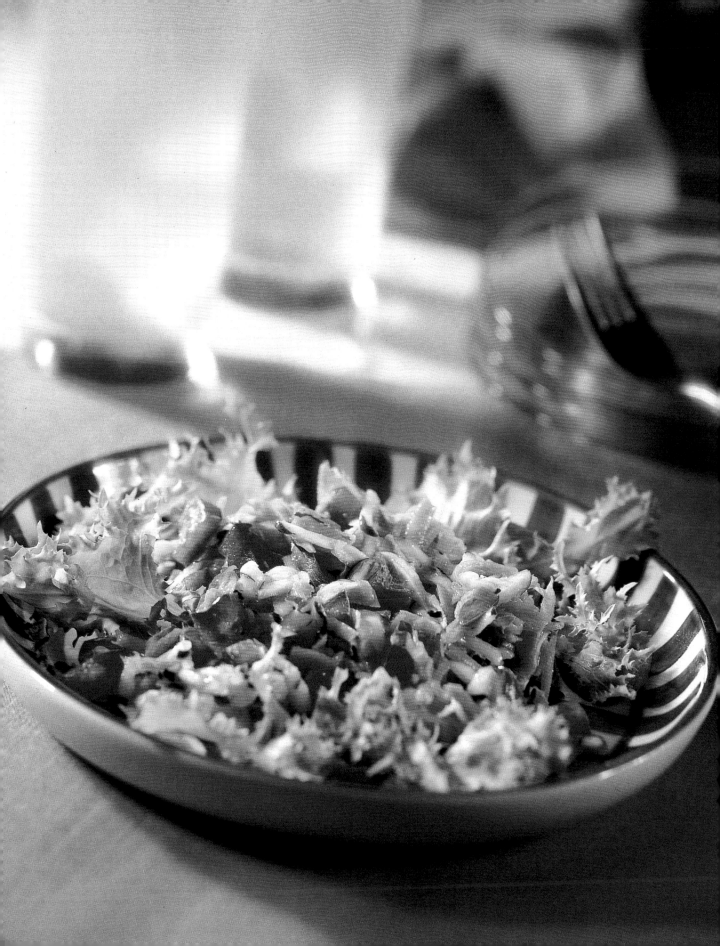

Poppy Seed Squash

PREP: 15 min; COOK: 7 min

4 SERVINGS

1 medium zucchini, cut into julienne strips

1 small yellow summer squash, cut into
    julienne strips

1 1/2 cups julienne strips jicama (6 ounces)

1 tablespoon cider or raspberry vinegar

1 tablespoon honey

1 teaspoon poppy seed

2 drops red pepper sauce

Place steamer basket in 1/2 inch water in saucepan
or skillet (water should not touch bottom of basket). Place zucchini, yellow squash and jicama in
basket. Cover tightly and heat to boiling; reduce
heat to low. Steam 3 to 5 minutes or until squash is
crisp-tender; drain. Place vegetables in serving
bowl. Mix remaining ingredients; drizzle over
vegetables.

1 Serving:		% Daily Value:	
Calories	35	Vitamin A	2%
Calories from fat	0	Vitamin C	12%
Fat, g	0	Calcium	2%
Saturated, g	0	Iron	4%
Cholesterol, mg	0	**Diet Exchanges:**	
Sodium, mg	5	2 vegetable	
Carbohydrate, g	11		
Dietary Fiber, g	3		
Protein, g	1		

Greek Salad

PREP: 10 min

4 SERVINGS

1 medium unpeeled cucumber

2 cups bite-size pieces spinach

2 cups bite-size pieces Boston lettuce

1/3 cup fat-free Caesar dressing

1/4 cup crumbled feta cheese

10 pitted ripe olives, sliced

1 medium tomato, cut into thin wedges

1 medium green onion, sliced
    (2 tablespoons)

Score cucumber by running tines of fork lengthwise down sides; slice. Toss cucumber and remaining ingredients.

1 Serving:		% Daily Value:	
Calories	65	Vitamin A	28%
Calories from fat	25	Vitamin C	30%
Fat, g	3	Calcium	10%
Saturated, g	3	Iron	8%
Cholesterol, mg	10	**Diet Exchanges:**	
Sodium, mg	430	2 vegetable	
Carbohydrate, g	8		
Dietary Fiber, g	2		
Protein, g	3		

Greek Salad

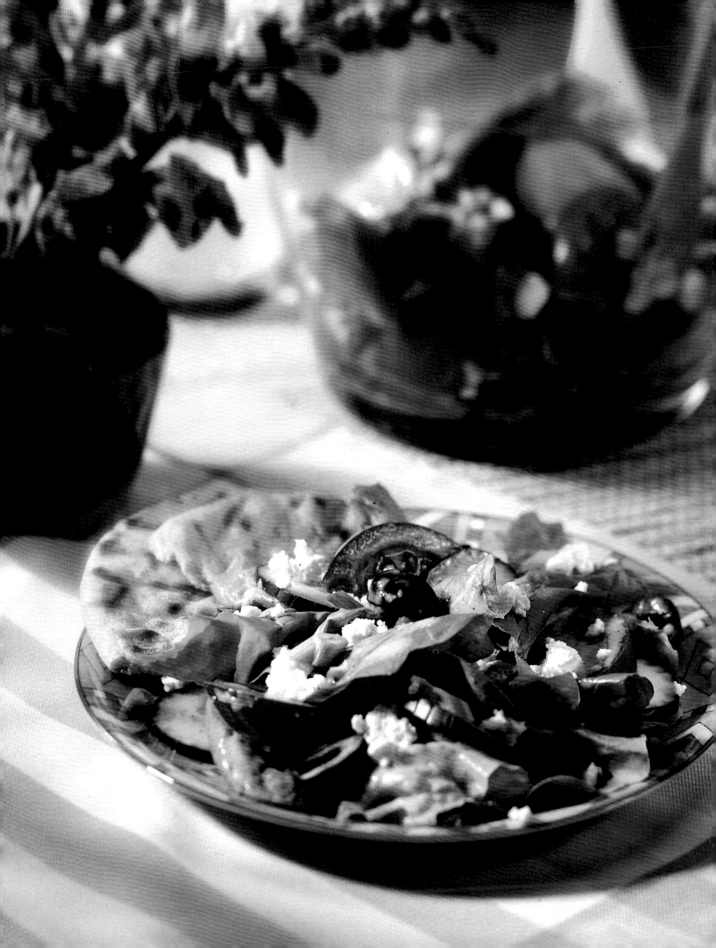

Blue Cheese Waldorf Salad

PREP: 15 min; CHILL: 1 hr

4 SERVINGS

Blue Cheese Dressing (below)

2 medium unpeeled red eating apples, cut into 1/4-inch slices

Lemon juice

Spinach leaves

1 medium stalk celery, thinly sliced (1/2 cup)

2 tablespoons chopped walnuts, toasted

Prepare Blue Cheese Dressing. Sprinkle apple slices with lemon juice. Place apple slices on spinach. Spoon dressing over salad. Sprinkle with celery and walnuts.

BLUE CHEESE DRESSING

1/3 cup plain fat-free yogurt

1 tablespoon fat-free mayonnaise or salad dressing

1 tablespoon finely crumbled blue cheese

Mix all ingredients. Cover and refrigerate at least 1 hour to blend flavors.

1 Serving:		% Daily Value:	
Calories	85	Vitamin A	8%
Calories from fat	25	Vitamin C	12%
Fat, g	3	Calcium	6%
Saturated, g	1	Iron	2%
Cholesterol, mg	2	**Diet Exchanges:**	
Sodium, mg	110	1 fruit	
Carbohydrate, g	14	1/2 fat	
Dietary Fiber, g	2		
Protein, g	2		

Crunchy Jicama and Melon Salad

PREP: 15 min; CHILL: 2 hr

6 SERVINGS

1 1/2 cups julienne strips jicama (6 ounces)

1/2 medium cantaloupe, cut into 1/2-inch cubes (1 1/2 cups)

2 tablespoons chopped fresh or 1 tablespoon dried mint leaves

1 teaspoon grated lime peel

3 tablespoons lime juice

1 teaspoon honey

1/4 teaspoon salt

Mix all ingredients in nonmetal bowl. Cover and refrigerate 2 hours to blend flavors.

1 Serving:		% Daily Value:	
Calories	45	Vitamin A	20%
Calories from fat	0	Vitamin C	76%
Fat, g	0	Calcium	2%
Saturated, g	0	Iron	2%
Cholesterol, mg	0	**Diet Exchanges:**	
Sodium, mg	110	1 fruit	
Carbohydrate, g	13		
Dietary Fiber, g	3		
Protein, g	1		

Asian Rice Salad

PREP: 10 min

4 SERVINGS

Sweet-and-sour dressing and bright vegetables make this a festive summer dish.

1/4 cup rice vinegar

1 1/2 teaspoons sugar or honey

1 teaspoon grated gingerroot

2 teaspoons sesame or vegetable oil

2 teaspoons reduced-sodium soy sauce or fish sauce

3 cups cooked white rice

1 small carrot, shredded (1/2 cup)

1/4 pound Chinese pea pods, strings removed and pea pods cut in half (1 cup)

Mix vinegar, sugar, gingerroot, oil and soy sauce in medium bowl. Stir in remaining ingredients.

1 Serving:		% Daily Value:	
Calories	195	Vitamin A	22%
Calories from fat	25	Vitamin C	22%
Fat, g	3	Calcium	2%
Saturated, g	0	Iron	12%
Cholesterol, mg	0	**Diet Exchanges:**	
Sodium, mg	110	2 starch/bread	
Carbohydrate, g	39	2 vegetable	
Dietary Fiber, g	1		
Protein, g	4		

Wild Rice and Pear Salad

PREP: 8 min

6 SERVINGS

Create a delicious main-dish salad by adding 1 to 2 cups of chopped smoked or regular turkey breast to this refreshing fruit and rice salad.

2 cups cooked wild rice

1/2 cup enoki or chopped regular white mushrooms

1/3 cup dried cranberries or raisins

1/3 cup fat-free red wine vinegar dressing

1 large pear, chopped

Mix all ingredients. Refrigerate at least 1 hour to blend flavors.

1 Serving:		% Daily Value:	
Calories	110	Vitamin A	0%
Calories from fat	0	Vitamin C	4%
Fat, g	0	Calcium	0%
Saturated, g	0	Iron	4%
Cholesterol, mg	0	**Diet Exchanges:**	
Sodium, mg	0	1 starch/bread	
Carbohydrate, g	26	1 vegetable	
Dietary Fiber, g	2	1/2 fruit	
Protein, g	3		

Tarragon Tomato Slices

PREP: 8 min; CHILL: 2 hr

6 SERVINGS

3 medium tomatoes, cut into 1/4-inch slices

1/4 cup tarragon wine vinegar or cider vinegar

1 tablespoon olive or vegetable oil

1 tablespoon chopped fresh or 1 teaspoon dried tarragon leaves

Freshly ground pepper

Lettuce leaves

Place tomatoes in nonmetal dish. Shake vinegar, oil and tarragon in tightly covered container; pour over tomatoes. Sprinkle with pepper. Cover and refrigerate at least 2 hours to blend flavors. Serve on lettuce.

1 Serving:		% Daily Value:	
Calories	35	Vitamin A	4%
Calories from fat	20	Vitamin C	20%
Fat, g	2	Calcium	0%
Saturated, g	0	Iron	2%
Cholesterol, mg	0	**Diet Exchanges:**	
Sodium, mg	5	1 vegetable	
Carbohydrate, g	4		
Dietary Fiber, g	1		
Protein, g	1		

Creamy Dilled Cucumbers

PREP: 8 min; CHILL: 4 hr

6 SERVINGS

1/2 cup plain fat-free yogurt

1 teaspoon chopped fresh or 1/4 teaspoon dried dill weed

1/2 teaspoon salt

1/8 teaspoon pepper

2 small peeled cucumbers, sliced (2 cups)

1 small red onion, thinly sliced and separated into rings

Mix all ingredients. Cover and refrigerate at least 4 hours to blend flavors.

1 Serving:		% Daily Value:	
Calories	25	Vitamin A	0%
Calories from fat	0	Vitamin C	6%
Fat, g	0	Calcium	4%
Saturated, g	0	Iron	0%
Cholesterol, mg	0	**Diet Exchanges:**	
Sodium, mg	210	1 vegetable	
Carbohydrate, g	4		
Dietary Fiber, g	0		
Protein, g	2		

PASS THE POTATOES PLEASE

You've probably heard this over and over again: Potatoes are fattening.

Not true! Complex carbohydrates such as potatoes, pasta, whole grains, fruits and vegetables do not make people fat. Loading potatoes up with butter or margarine, cream, sour cream, cheese or bacon is the fattening part, not the potato itself. Try topping potatoes with fat-free sour cream, plain fat-free yogurt, fat-free salad dressing, salsa or chopped fresh vegetables, herbs and fat-free Parmesan cheese.

There is no evidence that these foods increase your appetite and lead to more fat being stored in your body. Such claims may make the headlines, but cannot be supported with scientific facts.

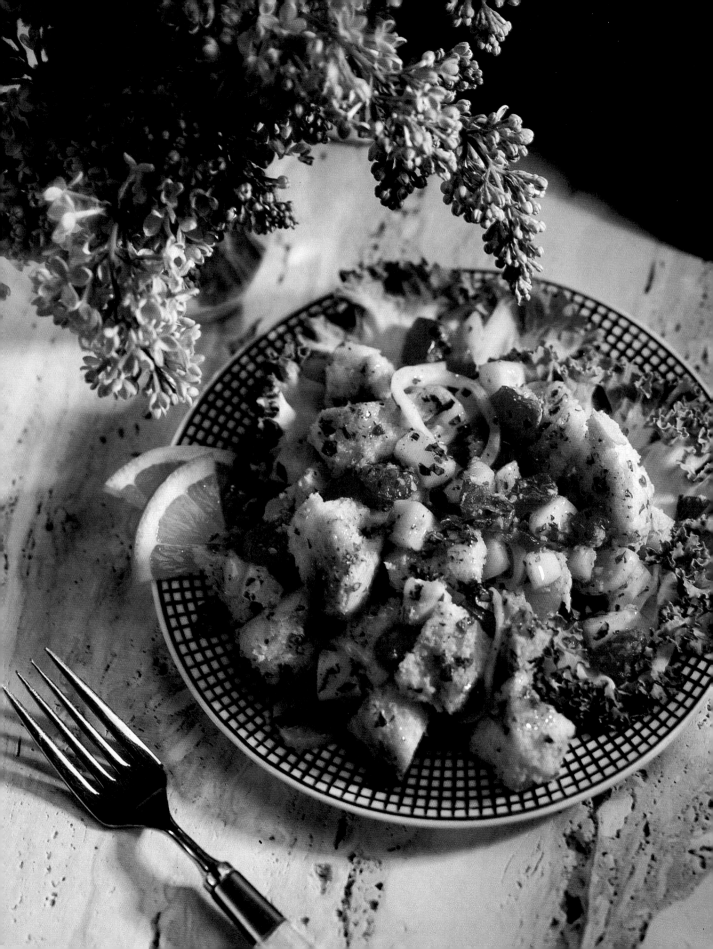

Bread Salad

PREP: 15 min

MAKES **6** SERVINGS

Making bread salad, or panzanella, *is a favorite way for Italian cooks to use up dried bread. It may turn into one of your favorites as well!*

6 one-inch slices day-old French or Italian bread

2 medium tomatoes, chopped (1 1/2 cups)

1 medium cucumber, peeled and chopped (1 1/4 cups)

1 small onion, thinly sliced

1/3 cup fat-free red wine vinegar dressing

2 tablespoons chopped fresh or 2 teaspoons dried basil leaves

1/4 teaspoon pepper

Tear bread into 1-inch pieces. Mix bread and remaining ingredients in nonmetal bowl. Cover and refrigerate, stirring once, at least 1 hour to blend flavors and soften bread. Stir before serving.

1 Serving:		% Daily Value:	
Calories	90	Vitamin A	4%
Calories from fat	10	Vitamin C	18%
Fat, g	1	Calcium	2%
Saturated, g	0	Iron	6%
Cholesterol, mg	0	**Diet Exchanges:**	
Sodium, mg	250	1 starch/bread	
Carbohydrate, g	18		
Dietary Fiber, g	1		
Protein, g	3		

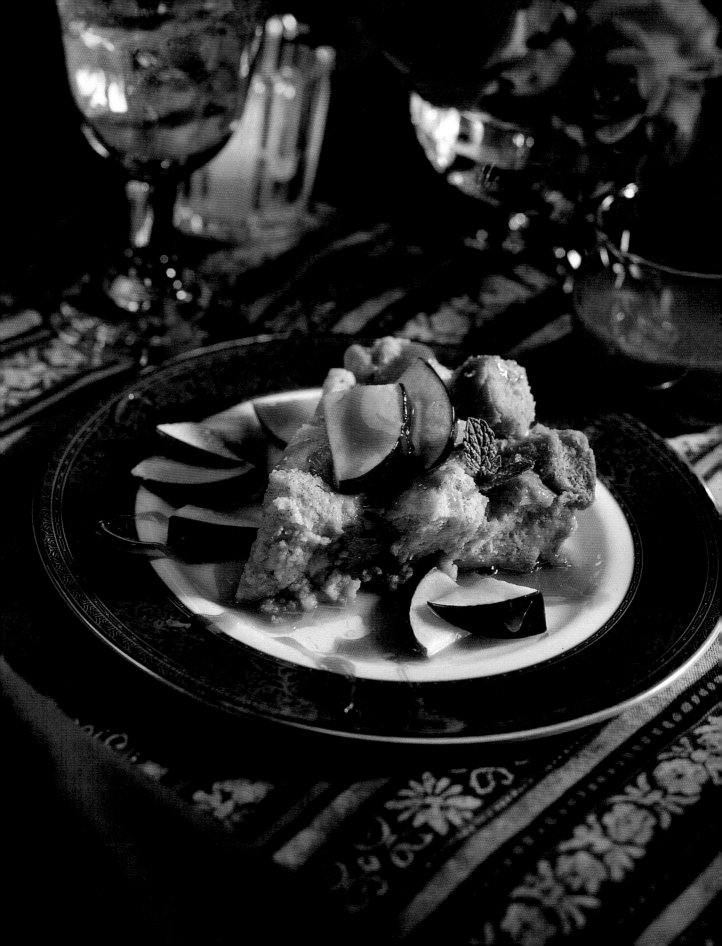

10

Desserts and Sweet Treats

Caramel-Apple Bread Pudding
(page 223)

Tira Mi Su Coffee Dessert

PREP: 10 min; CHILL: 1 hr

15 SERVINGS

Tiramisu is a rich coffee-flavored Italian dessert. The only drawback? It is typically high in fat. Our low-fat version comes to the rescue, and is just as delicious.

1 package (14 ounces) fat-free golden loaf cake, cut into 8 slices

1 cup strong coffee

1 package (8 ounces) reduced-fat cream cheese (Neufchâtel), softened

1/2 cup sugar

1/2 cup chocolate-flavored syrup

1 container (8 ounces) frozen reduced-fat whipped topping, thawed

Baking cocoa

Arrange cake slices to cover bottom of rectangular baking dish, 13 × 9 × 2 inches. Drizzle coffee over cake. Beat cream cheese, sugar and chocolate syrup in large bowl with electric mixer on medium speed until smooth. Gently stir in whipped topping until well blended. Spread over cake.

Cover and refrigerate about 1 hour or until set. Sprinkle with cocoa before serving. Cover and refrigerate any remaining dessert.

1 Serving:		% Daily Value:	
Calories	195	Vitamin A	4%
Calories from fat	55	Vitamin C	0%
Fat, g	6	Calcium	2%
Saturated, g	4	Iron	2%
Cholesterol, mg	10	**Diet Exchanges:**	
Sodium, mg	170	2 starch/bread	
Carbohydrate, g	32	1 fat	
Dietary Fiber, g	0		
Protein, g	3		

Easy Chocolate Cake with Broiled Topping

PREP: 10 min; BAKE: 32 min; BROIL: 2 min

8 SERVINGS

1 package Betty Crocker® Sweet Rewards® chocolate fat-free snack cake mix

1 cup water

2 egg whites or 1/4 cup fat-free cholesterol-free egg product

1/4 cup quick-cooking oats

1/4 cup packed brown sugar

2 tablespoons reduced-calorie spread or margarine

2 tablespoons coconut

2 tablespoons chopped pecans

Heat oven to 375°. Prepare and bake cake mix as directed on package, using water and egg whites. Meanwhile, mix oats and brown sugar in medium bowl. Cut in margarine, using pastry blender or crisscrossing 2 knives, until mixture is well blended. Stir in coconut and pecans. Sprinkle over hot cake.

Set oven control to broil. Broil cake with top 4 to 6 inches from heat 1 to 2 minutes or until topping is light golden brown. Serve warm.

1 Serving:		% Daily Value:	
Calories	245	Vitamin A	4%
Calories from fat	45	Vitamin C	0%
Fat, g	5	Calcium	6%
Saturated, g	1	Iron	4%
Cholesterol, mg	0	**Diet Exchanges:**	
Sodium, mg	450	3 starch/bread	
Carbohydrate, g	48		
Dietary Fiber, g	1		
Protein, g	3		

Easy Chocolate Cake with Broiled Topping

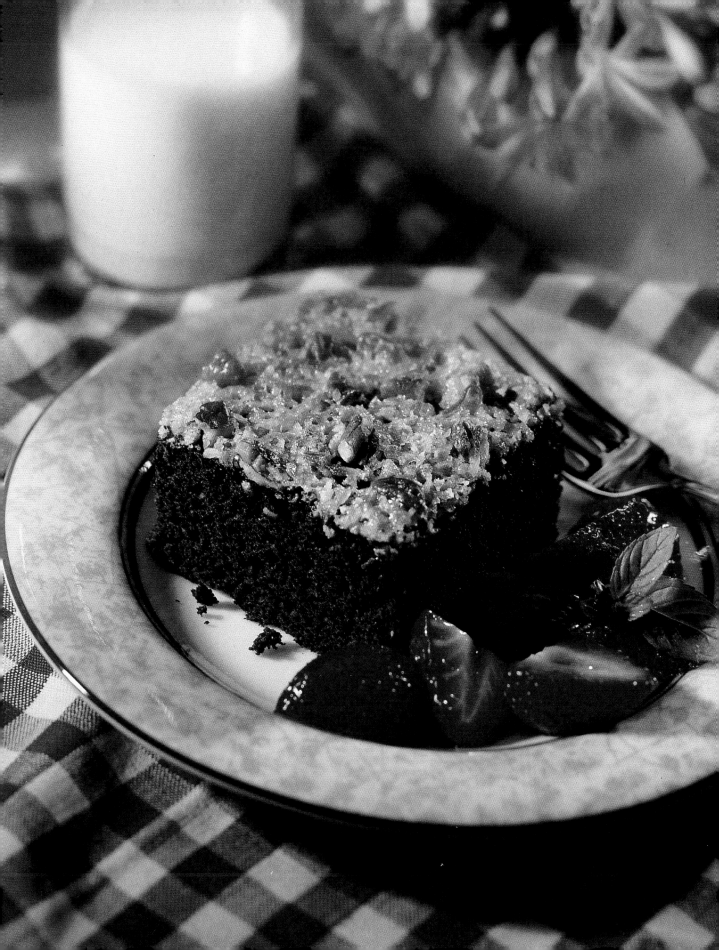

Banana-Caramel Pie

PREP: 15 min; CHILL: 3 hr

10 SERVINGS

Reduced-fat graham cracker pie crusts are now available at many stores. Using a reduced-fat crust lowers the fat and calories in this scrumptious pie even more. However, if one is not available, you'll still have a lower-fat pie if you use a regular pie crust recipe.

2 medium bananas, sliced

1 package (6 ounces) reduced-fat graham cracker pie crust

1 package (4-serving size) vanilla fat-free sugar-free instant pudding and pie filling

1 cup skim milk

2 cups frozen (thawed) reduced-fat whipped topping

1/4 cup caramel fat-free ice-cream topping

Place half of the banana slices in single layer in bottom of pie crust.

Beat pudding and pie filling (dry) and milk with wire whisk about 1 minute or until smooth. Fold in whipped topping. Spread half of the pudding mixture over bananas in pie crust. Top with remaining bananas. Spread with remaining pudding mixture. Cover and refrigerate about 3 hours or until set. Cut pie into wedges. Drizzle ice-cream topping over each serving. Cover and refrigerate any remaining pie.

1 Serving:		% Daily Value:	
Calories	190	Vitamin A	2%
Calories from fat	35	Vitamin C	4%
Fat, g	4	Calcium	4%
Saturated, g	3	Iron	0%
Cholesterol, mg	0	**Diet Exchanges:**	
Sodium, mg	230	2 1/2 starch/bread	
Carbohydrate, g	37		
Dietary Fiber, g	0		
Protein, g	2		

Caramel-Apple Bread Pudding

PREP: 15 min; BAKE: 45 min

8 SERVINGS

This dessert also makes a great breakfast—just use maple-flavored syrup or applesauce in place of the caramel ice-cream topping and serve with chopped fresh apples.

1 cup unsweetened applesauce

1/2 cup packed brown sugar

1 cup skim milk

1/2 cup fat-free cholesterol-free egg product

1 teaspoon vanilla

1/2 teaspoon ground cinnamon

5 cups 1-inch cubes French bread

1/2 cup caramel fat-free ice-cream topping, warmed

Heat oven to 350°. Spray quiche dish, 9 × 1 1/2 inches, or pie plate, 9 × 1 1/4 inches, with non-stick cooking spray. Mix all ingredients except bread and ice-cream topping in large bowl with wire whisk until smooth. Fold in bread. Pour into quiche dish.

Bake 40 to 45 minutes or until golden brown and set. Cut into wedges. Drizzle ice-cream topping over each serving.

1 Serving:		% Daily Value:	
Calories	190	Vitamin A	2%
Calories from fat	10	Vitamin C	0%
Fat, g	1	Calcium	6%
Saturated, g	0	Iron	6%
Cholesterol, mg	0	**Diet Exchanges:**	
Sodium, mg	155	1 starch/bread	
Carbohydrate, g	42	2 fruit	
Dietary Fiber, g	1		
Protein, g	4		

Raspberry Brûlée

PREP: 10 min; COOK: 10 min; BROIL: 3 min

8 SERVINGS

This dessert isn't just low-fat, it's easy! Crème brûlée, a restaurant favorite, can now be made quickly and deliciously at home.

1 cup raspberries

1/3 cup sugar

2 tablespoons cornstarch

1/4 teaspoon salt

2 cups fat-free half-and-half or skim milk

1/2 teaspoon vanilla

4 teaspoons packed brown sugar

Place raspberries evenly in bottom of four 10-ounce custard cups or ramekins. Mix sugar, cornstarch and salt in 2-quart saucepan. Stir in half-and-half. Heat to boiling over medium heat, stirring frequently. Stir in vanilla. Spoon over raspberries.

Set oven control to broil. Sprinkle 1 teaspoon brown sugar over mixture in each custard cup. Broil with tops 4 to 6 inches from heat 2 to 3 minutes or just until brown sugar is melted. Serve immediately. Cover and refrigerate any remaining desserts.

1 Serving:		% Daily Value:	
Calories	180	Vitamin A	8%
Calories from fat	0	Vitamin C	6%
Fat, g	0	Calcium	16%
Saturated, g	0	Iron	2%
Cholesterol, mg	2	**Diet Exchanges:**	
Sodium, mg	210	2 1/2 fruit	
Carbohydrate, g	43	1/2 skim milk	
Dietary Fiber, g	2		
Protein, g	4		

Raspberry Brûlée

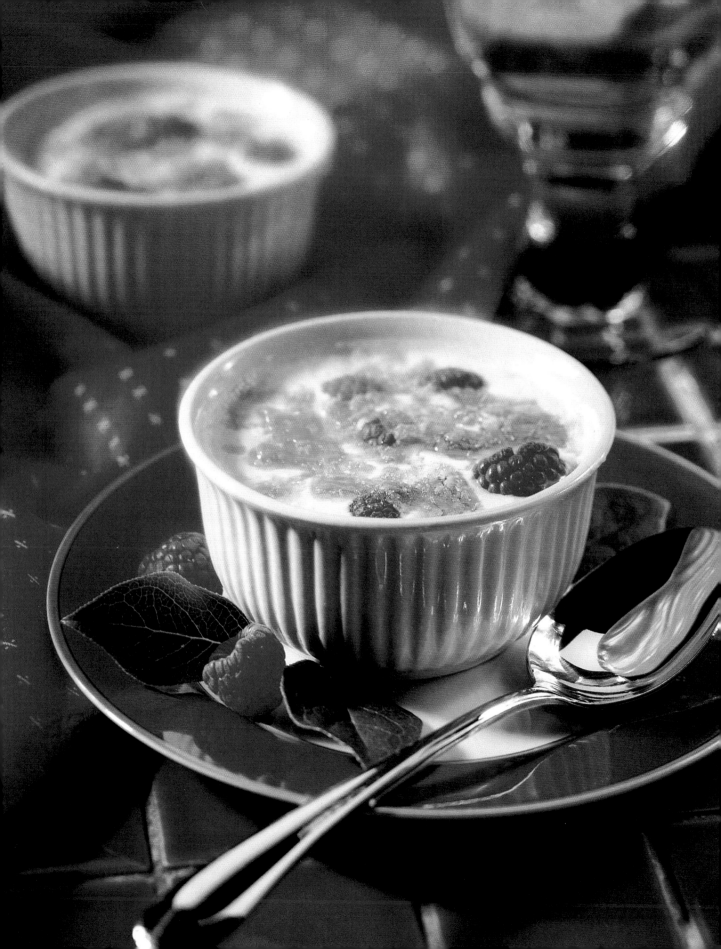

Maple Custard

PREP: **10 min**; BAKE: **45 min**; STAND: **15 min**

4 SERVINGS

1 egg

2 egg whites

3 tablespoons sugar

1/2 teaspoon maple flavoring

Dash of salt

1 3/4 cups very warm low-fat milk

4 teaspoons maple-flavored syrup

Heat oven to 350°. Beat egg, egg whites, sugar, maple flavoring and salt in medium bowl. Gradually stir in milk. Pour into four 6-ounce custard cups.

Drop 1 teaspoon maple syrup carefully onto center of mixture in each cup (syrup will sink to bottom). Place cups in square pan, 9 × 9 × 2 inches, on oven rack. Pour very hot water into pan to within 1/2 inch of tops of cups.

Bake about 45 minutes or until knife inserted halfway between center and edge comes out clean. Remove cups from water; let stand 15 minutes. Unmold, and serve warm. Or cover, refrigerate and unmold at serving time. Immediately cover and refrigerate any remaining custards.

1 Serving:		% Daily Value:	
Calories	135	Vitamin A	8%
Calories from fat	25	Vitamin C	0%
Fat, g	3	Calcium	14%
Saturated, g	2	Iron	0%
Cholesterol, mg	60	**Diet Exchanges:**	
Sodium, mg	180	1 fruit	
Carbohydrate, g	20	1/2 skim milk	
Dietary Fiber, g	0		
Protein, g	7		

Fat Substitutes for Baking

There is good news for home cooks who want to cut the fat. Because baking is really a science, in which exact ingredient combinations and amounts are critical, it is trickier to fight the fat monster, but it can be done. Fat contributes moistness and tenderness to baked goods and when there is not enough the results can be dry, tough, gummy or rubbery.

- Eggs and butter, margarine, oil or shortening are the primary sources of fat. Replacing whole eggs with cholesterol-free fat-free egg substitute or egg whites is easy. Replacing butter or margarine is more challenging. Applesauce, yogurt, pureed prunes and bananas as well as baby food all work, but none can be substituted for all of the fat in a recipe without sacrificing the taste, texture and appearance.

- Overall, applesauce and yogurt work the best in most recipes. They add the necessary moistness, don't alter the flavor as much as prunes and bananas do, and result in a good texture. The flavor of prune puree is especially good with chocolate, spice and carrot cakes. Banana puree works well in carrot and banana cake or muffins.

- Prune puree mixtures are now sold in the grocery store in the baking section; the label may state that it's a butter and oil or fat replacer (follow label directions for use).

- For best texture and flavor, we recommend replacing half of the fat (butter, margarine, shortening, oil) listed in a recipe with applesauce, yogurt, pureed prunes and bananas or baby food.

- Use cholesterol-free fat-free egg substitute or 2 egg whites for each whole egg called for in a recipe.

Look at the Savings

The original recipe calls for 1/2 cup margarine. The revised recipe uses 1/4 cup margarine and 1/4 cup applesauce. You have saved 400 calories and 44 grams of fat (the calories and fat in 1/4 cup margarine).

Pumpkin-Molasses Cheesecakes

PREP: 10 min; BAKE: 35 min

8 SERVINGS

2 soft molasses cookies (3 inches in diameter)

1 package (8 ounces) fat-free cream cheese, softened

1/3 cup packed brown sugar

1/2 cup fat-free cholesterol-free egg product

1/2 teaspoon vanilla

2/3 cup canned pumpkin

1/2 teaspoon pumpkin pie spice

1 cup frozen (thawed) reduced-fat whipped topping

Heat oven to 350°. Line 8 medium muffin cups, 2 1/2 × 1 1/4 inches, with foil or paper baking cups. Break cookies into fine crumbs. Reserve 2 teaspoons cookie crumbs for topping. Divide remaining crumbs among muffin cups.

Beat cream cheese and brown sugar in medium bowl with electric mixer on medium speed until smooth. Using spoon, stir in egg product and vanilla just until blended. Stir in pumpkin and pumpkin pie spice. Spoon evenly into muffin cups.

Bake 30 to 35 minutes or until edges are set. Refrigerate until completely chilled (centers will sink while cooling). Serve each cheesecake topped with 2 tablespoons whipped topping. Sprinkle with reserved cookie crumbs. Sprinkle with pumpkin pie spice if desired. Cover and refrigerate any remaining cheesecakes.

1 Serving:		% Daily Value:	
Calories	100	Vitamin A	46%
Calories from fat	20	Vitamin C	0%
Fat, g	2	Calcium	4%
Saturated, g	2	Iron	4%
Cholesterol, mg	0	**Diet Exchanges:**	
Sodium, mg	210	1/2 fruit	
Carbohydrate, g	16	1/2 skim milk	
Dietary Fiber, g	1		
Protein, g	6		

Pumpkin-Molasses Cheesecakes

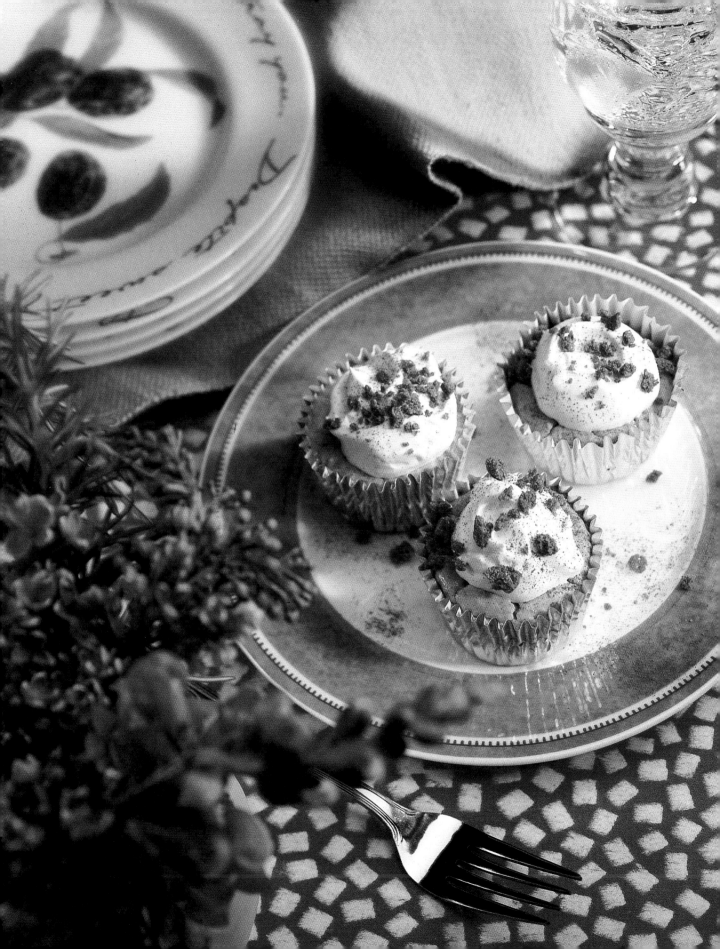

SHOPPING SMART

- Never shop when you're hungry.

- Use a grocery list and stick to it.

- Become an avid label reader so you know what you're paying for.

- Look for products that are reduced in fat and calories or fat-free.

- Buy healthful snacks such as fat-free pretzels, flavored rice cakes and popcorn cakes, and indulge in the purchase of prewashed, precut vegetables—they're so easy to grab and eat or to take with you. This will help to prevent sabotaging good intentions.

- Buy healthful desserts such as low-fat or fat-free yogurt or ice cream and frozen yogurt.

- Follow the golden rule: If you don't buy it, you can't eat it!

Crunchy Pears

PREP: 15 min; BAKE: 45 min

4 SERVINGS

4 firm ripe large pears
1/4 cup orange juice
3 tablespoons orange marmalade
3 tablespoons vanilla wafer crumbs
3 tablespoons chopped almonds
1/2 cup orange or plain fat-free yogurt
Cinnamon, if desired

Move oven rack to lowest position. Heat oven to 350°. Spray pie plate, 9 × 1 1/4 inches, with non-stick cooking spray. Carefully peel pears, leaving stems attached; place on large plate. Mix orange juice and marmalade; spoon over pears.

Mix wafer crumbs and almonds. Roll pears in crumb mixture; stand pears upright in pie plate. Mix yogurt and remaining marmalade mixture from plate; refrigerate. Bake pears 35 to 45 minutes or until tender when pierced with fork (baking time may vary due to size of pears). Serve warm with yogurt sauce and sprinkle with cinnamon.

1 Serving:		% Daily Value:	
Calories	245	Vitamin A	2%
Calories from fat	35	Vitamin C	14%
Fat, g	4	Calcium	8%
Saturated, g	1	Iron	6%
Cholesterol, mg	0	**Diet Exchanges:**	
Sodium, mg	25	1 starch/bread	
Carbohydrate, g	55	2 1/2 fruit	
Dietary Fiber, g	6		
Protein, g	3		

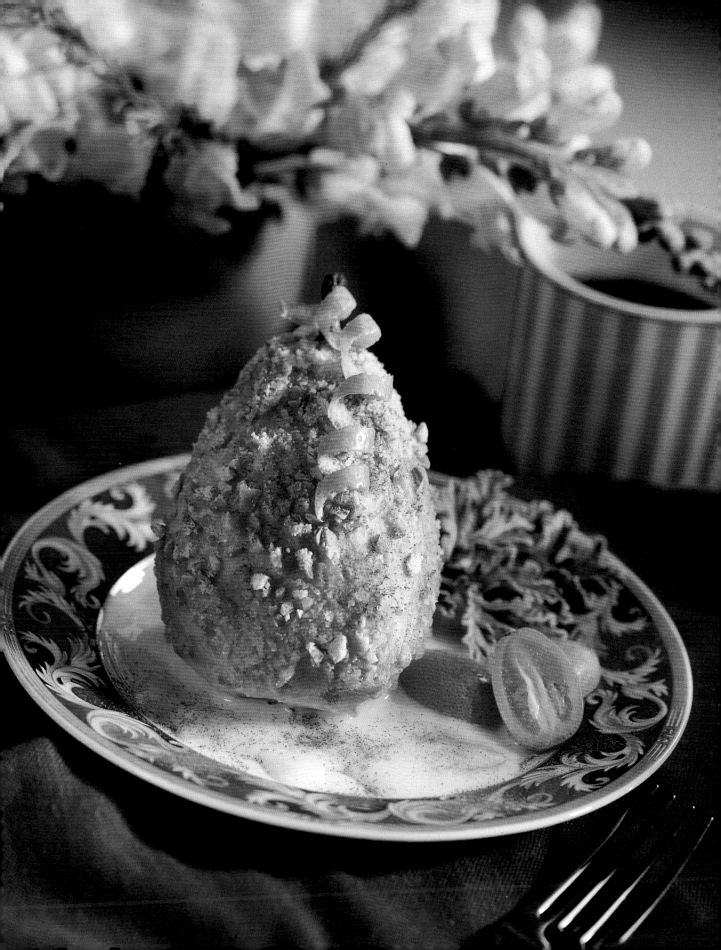

Raspberry-Graham Cracker Torte

PREP: 15 min; CHILL: 12 hr

6 SERVINGS

1 cup raspberries

1/2 teaspoon almond extract

2 1/2 cups frozen (thawed) reduced-fat whipped topping

7 graham cracker rectangles, 5 × 2 1/2 inches each (about 3/4 packet)

Place raspberries in food processor or blender. Cover and process until smooth; reserve 1/4 cup. Cover and refrigerate. Fold remaining raspberry puree and the almond extract into whipped topping until creamy.

Spread 1 cracker with about 2 tablespoons topping mixture; layer with a second cracker. Place on serving plate. Repeat layers 5 times. Gently press torte together. Using pancake turner, carefully turn torte on its side so crackers are on long sides. Frost top and sides with remaining topping mixture.

Cover and refrigerate at least 12 hours or overnight (torte will soften and crackers will become moist). Serve torte with reserved raspberry puree. Cover and refrigerate any remaining torte.

1 Serving:		% Daily Value:	
Calories	130	Vitamin A	0%
Calories from fat	45	Vitamin C	8%
Fat, g	5	Calcium	2%
Saturated, g	4	Iron	4%
Cholesterol, mg	2	**Diet Exchanges:**	
Sodium, mg	120	1 starch/bread	
Carbohydrate, g	21	1/2 fruit	
Dietary Fiber, g	2	1 fat	
Protein, g	2		

Creamy Strawberry Angel Cake

PREP: 20 min; CHILL: 1 1/4 hr

12 SERVINGS

1 cup boiling water

1 package (4-serving size) strawberry-flavored sugar-free gelatin

1/2 cup cold water

1 pint strawberries (2 cups)

1 container (8 ounces) frozen reduced-fat whipped topping, thawed

10-inch round angel food cake

Pour boiling water on gelatin in large bowl; stir until gelatin is dissolved. Stir in cold water. Refrigerate about 1 hour or until thickened but not set.

Slice strawberries, reserving a few whole berries for garnish if desired. Fold sliced strawberries and half of the whipped topping into gelatin. Refrigerate about 15 minutes or until thickened but not set.

Split cake horizontally to make 3 layers. (To split, mark side of cake with toothpicks and cut with long, thin serrated knife.) Fill layers with gelatin mixture. Spread remaining whipped topping over top. Garnish with whole strawberries. Cut with long, thin serrated knife. Cover and refrigerate any remaining cake.

1 Serving:		% Daily Value:	
Calories	195	Vitamin A	0%
Calories from fat	25	Vitamin C	22%
Fat, g	3	Calcium	2%
Saturated, g	2	Iron	4%
Cholesterol, mg	0	**Diet Exchanges:**	
Sodium, mg	400	1 starch/bread	
Carbohydrate, g	38	1 1/2 fruit	
Dietary Fiber, g	0		
Protein, g	4		

Strawberry Pie with Meringue Crust

PREP: 15 min; BAKE: 40 min;
STAND: 1 hr; CHILL: 1 hr

8 SERVINGS

2 egg whites

1/8 teaspoon cream of tartar

1/4 cup sugar

**1 package (1.1 ounces) vanilla fat-free sugar-
free instant pudding and pie filling**

1 cup skim milk

**1 1/2 cups frozen (thawed) reduced-fat
whipped topping**

1 pint strawberries (2 cups), sliced

Heat oven to 275°. Spray pie plate, 9 × 1 1/4
inches, with nonstick cooking spray. Beat egg
whites and cream of tartar in medium bowl with
electric mixer on high speed until foamy. Beat in
sugar, 1 tablespoon at a time; continue beating
until stiff and glossy. Do not underbeat. Spread
mixture evenly on bottom and halfway up side of
pie plate. Bake 40 minutes. Turn off oven; leave
meringue in oven with door closed 1 hour. Finish
cooling meringue at room temperature.

Beat pudding and pie filling (dry) and milk about
45 seconds, using wire whisk. Fold in 1 cup of the
whipped topping. Layer half of the pudding mixture and half of the strawberries in crust; repeat.

Cover loosely and refrigerate until firm, at least
1 hour but no longer than 8 hours. Run knife
around edge to loosen crust. Top each serving with
some of the remaining 1/2 cup whipped topping.
Cover and refrigerate any remaining pie.

1 Serving:		% Daily Value:	
Calories	85	Vitamin A	2%
Calories from fat	20	Vitamin C	36%
Fat, g	2	Calcium	4%
Saturated, g	2	Iron	0%
Cholesterol, mg	0	**Diet Exchanges:**	
Sodium, mg	180	1 fruit	
Carbohydrate, g	16		
Dietary Fiber, g	1		
Protein, g	2		

Pear-Date Streusel Bars

PREP: 10 min; BAKE: 45 min

36 BARS

Old-fashioned date bars with a twist—less fat and filled with a moist pear and date filling.

1 can (16 ounces) pear halves in extra-light syrup, drained and juice reserved

1 package (8 ounces) chopped dates

1 cup all-purpose flour

1 cup quick-cooking oats

3/4 cup packed brown sugar

1/2 teaspoon baking soda

1/4 teaspoon salt

1/2 cup reduced-calorie spread or margarine

Powdered sugar, if desired

Finely chop pears. Heat pears, reserved pear juice and the dates to boiling in 2-quart saucepan over medium-high heat; reduce heat to low. Cook uncovered, stirring occasionally, until thickened. Cool slightly.

Heat oven to 350°. Spray rectangular pan, 13 × 9 inches, with nonstick cooking spray. Mix flour, oats, brown sugar, baking soda and salt in large bowl. Cut in margarine, using pastry blender or crisscrossing 2 knives, until mixture resembles fine crumbs. Reserve 1 cup of crumbly mixture for topping. Press remaining mixture in bottom of pan. Bake 15 minutes.

Carefully spread date mixture over crust. Sprinkle with remaining crumbly mixture; press lightly. Bake about 30 minutes or until light golden brown. Cool completely. Sprinkle with powdered sugar. Cut into 2 × 1 1/2-inch bars.

1 Bar:		% Daily Value:	
Calories	85	Vitamin A	4%
Calories from fat	25	Vitamin C	0%
Fat, g	3	Calcium	0%
Saturated, g	1	Iron	2%
Cholesterol, mg	0	**Diet Exchanges:**	
Sodium, mg	65	1 starch/bread	
Carbohydrate, g	15		
Dietary Fiber, g	1		
Protein, g	1		

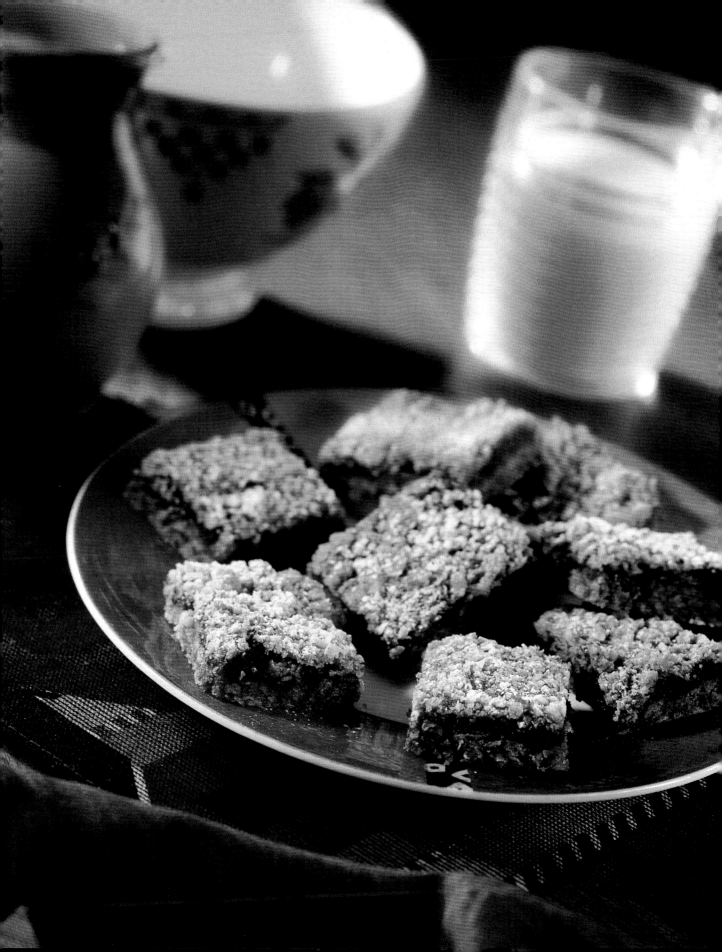

Honeydew Sorbet with Strawberry Purée

PREP: 10 min; FREEZE: 2 hr

6 SERVINGS

**1/2 medium honeydew melon, peeled and
cut into 1-inch chunks**

1 pint strawberries (2 cups)

1 teaspoon lemon juice

6 whole strawberries

Place melon chunks in ungreased jelly roll pan, 15 1/2 × 10 1/2 × 1 inch. Cover and freeze at least 2 hours until hardened.

Place 1 pint strawberries in food processor. Cover and process until smooth. Place about 3 tablespoons strawberry purée on each of 6 dessert plates.

Wash and dry workbowl of food processor. Place half of the frozen melon chunks and 1/2 teaspoon of the lemon juice in food processor. Cover and process until smooth. Repeat with remaining melon and lemon juice. Scoop or spoon about 1/2 cup melon mixture over strawberry purée on each plate. (Melon mixture may be frozen up to 30 minutes before serving.) Garnish with whole strawberries. Serve immediately.

Note: If sorbet is frozen, allow it to stand at room temperature about 30 to 45 minutes to soften.

1 Serving:		% Daily Value:	
Calories	60	Vitamin A	0%
Calories from fat	0	Vitamin C	100%
Fat, g	0	Calcium	2%
Saturated, g	0	Iron	2%
Cholesterol, mg	0	**Diet Exchanges:**	
Sodium, mg	10	1 fruit	
Carbohydrate, g	14		
Dietary Fiber, g	2		
Protein, g	1		

Chocolate Chip Cookies

PREP: 10 min; BAKE: 10 min

ABOUT 4 1/2 DOZEN COOKIES

Yes, you can enjoy your favorite cookies and stay on your diet!

1/2 cup granulated sugar

1/4 cup packed brown sugar

1/4 cup margarine, softened

1 teaspoon vanilla

1 egg white or 2 tablespoons fat-free cholesterol-free egg product

1 cup all-purpose flour

1/2 teaspoon baking soda

1/4 teaspoon salt

1/2 cup miniature semisweet chocolate chips

Heat oven to 375°. Mix sugars, margarine, vanilla and egg white in large bowl. Stir in flour, baking soda and salt. Stir in chocolate chips.

Drop dough by rounded teaspoonfuls about 2 inches apart onto ungreased cookie sheet. Bake 8 to 10 minutes or until golden brown. Cool slightly; remove from cookie sheet to wire rack.

1 Cookie:		% Daily Value:	
Calories	60	Vitamin A	2%
Calories from fat	20	Vitamin C	0%
Fat, g	2	Calcium	0%
Saturated, g	1	Iron	2%
Cholesterol, mg	0	**Diet Exchanges:**	
Sodium, mg	60	1 1/2 starch/bread	
Carbohydrate, g	10		
Dietary Fiber, g	0		
Protein, g	1		

Menus for Two Weeks

Meal and menu planning can be difficult and time-consuming, particularly if you are trying to lose weight. Average recommended caloric intake for healthy adults is 2,000 calories and 65 grams of fat per day.[1] Your needs may be higher or lower depending on your height, frame, gender and activity level. If you are trying to lose weight, you will want to decrease your calorie and fat intake and increase your activity level.

The menus in this section will help you choose a variety of foods that meet a reduced calorie and fat eating plan. These menus vary from 1,345 to 1,625 calories and 21 to 39 grams of fat per day. You don't have to follow these menus in any particular order. You are free to mix and match meal menus from different days to add variety to your eating plan. Just keep track of your total calories and grams of fat to assure you're not eating too much or too little. It's that simple. It's up to you.

[1]*Nutrition Facts, Food and Drug Administration, 1994.*

Menu 1

BREAKFAST

1 serving Mother Earth Pancakes (page 58)

1/4 cup light maple-flavored syrup

1/2 cup blueberries

1 cup skim milk

Calories 335 • Fat 1g • Fiber 1g

LUNCH

1 carton (6 ounces) nonfat yogurt, any flavor

1 bagel

1 tablespoon Neufachâtel cream cheese

1/2 cup potato salad or coleslaw

1 cup sliced strawberries

Calories 505 • Fat 16g • Fiber 6g

DINNER

1 serving Savory Chicken and Rice (page 104)

1 cup cooked broccoli

1 dinner roll

1/2 cup mixed fresh fruit

1/2 cup frozen fruit-flavored sorbet

Calories 605 • Fat 7g • Fiber 10g

SNACK

1 Chocolate Chip Cookie (page 237)

1 cup skim milk

Calories 150 • Fat 3g • Fiber 0g

TOTAL: CALORIES 1595 • FAT 27g • FIBER 20g

Menu 2

BREAKFAST

1 serving Herbed Eggs with Salsa (page 52)

2 slices whole wheat toast

2 teaspoons jam or jelly

1/2 medium grapefruit

1 cup skim milk

Calories 390 • Fat 5g • Fiber 7g

LUNCH

1 cup tomato soup (made with skim milk)

1 Tomato-Basil Biscuit (page 201)

1/2 cup marinated vegetable salad

1 kiwifruit, sliced

Calories 450 • Fat 20g • Fiber 6g

DINNER

1 serving Meat Loaf (page 130)

1 small baked potato

2 tablespoons reduced-fat sour cream

1 1/2 cups cooked frozen broccoli, cauliflower
and carrots

Tossed salad

2 tablespoons fat-free dressing

1/2 cup sugar-free chocolate pudding
made with skim milk

Calories 395 • Fat 10g • Fiber 10g

SNACK

2 cups 94% fat-free microwave popcorn

1/2 cup cran-raspberry juice

Calories 115 • Fat 1g • Fiber 1g

TOTAL: CALORIES 1350 • FAT 36g • FIBER 24g

Menu 3

BREAKFAST

1 serving Wake-Up Shake (page 59)

1 cup pineapple chunks

Calories 290 • Fat 1g • Fiber 6g

LUNCH

Tuna sandwich made with 2 ounces water-packed tuna mixed with 2 teaspoons mayonnaise or salad dressing and 1 teaspoon Dijon mustard

2 slices whole wheat or white bread

10 reduced-fat potato chips

1 medium dill pickle

1 cup skim milk

Calories 445 • Fat 15g • Fiber 5g

DINNER

1 serving Garden-Fresh Primavera (page 160)

1 sourdough or hard roll

2 teaspoons margarine

1 slice (1/12th of round cake) angel food cake

1/2 cup sliced strawberries

2 tablespoons non-dairy whipped topping

Calories 635 • Fat 13g • Fiber 2g

SNACK

1 peach or nectarine

1/2 cup frozen low-fat yogurt

Calories 135 • Fat 1g • Fiber 2g

TOTAL: CALORIES 1505 • FAT 33g • FIBER 20g

Menu 4

BREAKFAST

1 serving Stuffed French Toast (page 58)

1/2 cup orange juice

Calories 315 • Fat 5g • Fiber 2g

LUNCH

1 cup vegetarian bean soup

6 soda crackers

1 ounce American cheese reduced-fat spread

3/4 cup grapes

1 cup skim milk

Calories 590 • Fat 15g • Fiber 4g

DINNER

1 serving Chicken-Fusilli-Vegetable Toss (page 152)

Mixed green salad

2 tablespoons fat-free dressing

1 petite pan or hard roll

1 teaspoon margarine

1 frozen gelatin pop

Calories 485 • Fat 15g • Fiber 4g

SNACK

4 graham cracker squares

3/4 cup melon chunks

1 cup skim milk

Calories 235 • Fat 3g • Fiber 1g

TOTAL: CALORIES 1625 • FAT 39g • FIBER 25g

Menu 5

....

BREAKFAST

1 serving Morning Parfaits (page 60)

1 English Muffin

2 teaspoons reduced-fat peanut butter spread

Calories 345 • Fat 9g • Fiber 4g

LUNCH

2 ounces fat-free smoked or regular turkey slices
rolled in one (8-inch) flour tortilla with
1/3 cup shredded lettuce, 2 tablespoons shredded
reduced-fat Cheddar cheese and 2 tablespoons salsa

1/2 cup vegetarian baked beans

1 apple

Calories 410 • Fat 8g • Fiber 12g

DINNER

1 serving Chicken Breast Dijon (page 96)

1 cup cooked asparagus

3/4 cup cooked couscous

2 plums

1 cup skim milk

Calories 495 • Fat 7g • Fiber 8g

SNACK

1 ounce pretzels

1 cup chocolate skim milk

Calories 245 • Fat 3g • Fiber 4g

....

TOTAL: CALORIES 1495 • FAT 27g • FIBER 28g

Menu 6

....

BREAKFAST

1 serving Lemon Muesli (page 54)

1/2 cup blueberries

1 rice cake

1 teaspoon margarine

Calories 395 • Fat 7g • Fiber 7g

LUNCH

1 cup chicken noodle soup

1 serving Dill Casserole Bread (page 201)

Carrot and celery sticks

1 medium pear

1 cup skim milk

Calories 430 • Fat 8g • Fiber 8g

DINNER

1 serving Red Snapper with Tropical Relish (page 114)

1 cup cooked green beans

3/4 cup mashed potatoes

Tossed salad

2 tablespoons fat-free dressing

1 apricot

Calories 395 • Fat 11g • Fiber 10g

SNACK

3/4 cup sherbet

Calories 205 • Fat 3g • Fiber 0g

....

TOTAL: CALORIES 1425 • FAT 29g • FIBER 25g

Menu 7

BREAKFAST

1 Lemon–Poppy Seed Scone (page 63)

1 carton (6 ounces) nonfat yogurt, any flavor

1/2 cup cranberry juice

Calories 415 • Fat 9g • Fiber 0g

LUNCH

1 ounce thin slice ham

1 ounce reduced-fat American or
Swiss cheese slice

2 slices pumpernickel or rye bread

1 teaspoon margarine

1 cup tomato soup (made with skim milk)

1 cup baby carrots

Calories 455 • Fat 15g • Fiber 8g

DINNER

1 serving Stir-Fried Garlic Shrimp (page 126)

1 cup cooked frozen sugar snap peas,
cauliflower and carrots

1 cup cooked rice

1 orange

Calories 515 • Fat 5g • Fiber 8g

SNACK

1/2 cup frozen fat-free yogurt or ice cream

1 tablespoon fat-free chocolate fudge
ice cream topping

Calories 155 • Fat 0g • Fiber 0g

TOTAL: CALORIES 1540 • FAT 29g • FIBER 16g

Menu 8

BREAKFAST

1 serving Banana-Peach Shake (page 59)

1 scrambled egg

1 Mango-Lime Muffin (page 63)

Calories 335 • Fat 9g • Fiber 3g

LUNCH

1 fat-free hot dog

1 hot dog bun

1 tablespoon chopped onion

2 teaspoons sweet pickle relish

2 teaspoons catsup or mustard

10 reduced-fat potato chips

1 orange

Calories 325 • Fat 7g • Fiber 5g

DINNER

1 serving Risotto Primavera (page 176)

Mixed green salad with hard-cooked egg

2 tablespoons fat-free salad dressing

1 hard breadstick

1 teaspoon margarine

1 cup melon cubes

1 Pear-Date Streusel Bar (page 234)

1 cup skim milk

Calories 495 • Fat 13g • Fiber 7g

SNACK

1 cup Savory Popcorn Mix (page 46)

1/2 cup apple cider

Calories 190 • Fat 6g • Fiber 1g

TOTAL: CALORIES 1345 • FAT 35g • FIBER 16g

Menu 9

BREAKFAST

1 serving Fresh Fruit Bruschetta (page 60)

1 cup skim milk

1/2 cup orange or grapefruit juice

Calories 260 • Fat 1g • Fiber 2g

LUNCH

1 serving Raspberry-Chicken Salad (page 76)

1 small crusty dinner roll

1 teaspoon margarine

1 cup grapes

1 cup skim milk

Calories 510 • Fat 11g • Fiber 7g

DINNER

1 serving Swiss Steak (page 130)

1 medium baked potato

1 teaspoon margarine

1/2 cup corn

Carrot-raisin salad made with 1/2 cup shredded carrots, 1 tablespoon raisins and 2 teaspoons mayonnaise or salad dressing

1 nectarine or peach

Calories 540 • Fat 18g • Fiber 9g

SNACK

3 cups 94% fat-free microwave popcorn

Calories 60 • Fat 1g • Fiber 2g

TOTAL: CALORIES 1370 • FAT 31g • FIBER 20g

Menu 10

BREAKFAST

1/2 cup bran shreds cereal

1 slice toast with 1 teaspoon margarine, 1 teaspoon sugar and 1/8 teaspoon cinnamon

1 cup skim milk

1/2 banana

Calories 320 • Fat 7g • Fiber 14g

LUNCH

1 serving Creamy Vegetable-Cheese Soup (page 70)

1 bagel

1 tablespoon reduced-fat peanut butter spread

1/2 cup pineapple chunks

1 cup skim milk

Calories 500 • Fat 9g • Fiber 4g

DINNER

1 serving Grilled Southwestern Pork Chops (page 142)

1 cup grilled zucchini and yellow summer squash

1/2 cup noodles tossed with 1 tablespoon fat-free Italian dressing

1 medium tomato, sliced

1/2 cup applesauce

Calories 415 • Fat 10g • Fiber 5g

SNACK

1 serving Easy Chocolate Cake with Broiled Topping (page 220)

Calories 245 • Fat 5g • Fiber 1g

TOTAL: CALORIES 1480 • FAT 31g • FIBER 24g

Menu 11

Breakfast

3/4 cup hot oatmeal (made with skim milk)

2 teaspoons brown sugar

1 tablespoon raisins

1/2 grapefruit

1 cup skim milk

Calories 345 • Fat 3g • Fiber 5g

Lunch

1 serving Roast Beef Pocket Sandwiches
(page 86)

1 serving Black Bean and Corn Salad
(page 183)

10 reduced-fat baked tortilla chips

2 tablespoons Almost Guacamole (page 32)

Calories 380 • Fat 4g • Fiber 11g

Dinner

Spicy Couscous with Chilies and Vegetables
(page 192)

Tossed salad with 2 tablespoons reduced-fat
shredded Cheddar cheese

2 tablespoons fat-free dressing

1 serving Raspberry Brûlée (page 224)

1 cup skim milk

Calories 560 • Fat 6g • Fiber 9g

Snack

1 serving Irish Yogurt Bread (page 202)

1 teaspoon margarine

1 teaspoon jam or jelly

Calories 225 • Fat 8g • Fiber 1g

TOTAL: CALORIES 1510 • FAT 21g • FIBER 26g

Menu 12

Breakfast

1 scrambled egg

1 slice raisin bread, toasted

2 teaspoons jam or jelly

1 cup skim milk

1/2 cup cranberry juice

Calories 345 • Fat 7g • Fiber 1g

Lunch

1 serving Chunky Chili Soup (page 70)

1 corn muffin

1/2 cup canned mixed fruit or fruit cocktail

1 cup skim milk

Calories 470 • Fat 12g • Fiber 6g

Dinner

1 serving Pork with Basil (page 140)

1 cup rice

1/2 cup cooked bell pepper strips

1 small cucumber, sliced, with 2 teaspoons sugar
and 1 tablespoon vinegar

1 serving Tira Mi Su Coffee Dessert (page 220)

Calories 545 • Fat 11g • Fiber 3g

Snack

1 small apple

1 cup Southwestern Popcorn Snack (page 46)

Calories 145 • Fat 4g • Fiber 5g

TOTAL: CALORIES 1505 • FAT 34g • FIBER 15g

Menu 13

BREAKFAST

1 Lemon-Filled Fresh Ginger Scone (page 65)

1 carton (6 ounces) nonfat yogurt, any flavor

1/2 cup blueberries

Calories 42 • Fat 10g • Fiber 3g

LUNCH

1 serving Beef-Macaroni Salad (page 78)

1 Carrot-Zucchini Muffin (page 202)

1 teaspoon margarine

1/2 cup fresh cherries

1 cup skim milk

Calories 525 • Fat 11g • Fiber 5g

DINNER

2 servings Roasted-Vegetable Pizza (page 168)

Tossed salad

2 tablespoons fat-free dressing

1 sugar-free popsicle

Calories 435 • Fat 12g • Fiber 7g

SNACK

1 medium pear

Calories 95 • Fat 1g • Fiber 4g

TOTAL: CALORIES 1480 • FAT 34g • FIBER 19g

Menu 14

BREAKFAST

1 serving Vegetable-Egg Fajitas (page 53)

1 cup skim milk

1/2 cup pineapple juice

Calories 380 • Fat 4g • Fiber 3g

LUNCH

1 serving Pita Pizzas (page 171)

1/4 honeydew melon

1 cup skim milk

Calories 555 • Fat 8g • Fiber 12g

DINNER

1 serving Garlic Chicken Kiev (page 94)

1 cup cooked bell pepper strips

Caesar salad made with 1 cup romaine lettuce, 1 tablespoon reduced-fat Caesar salad dressing and 1 tablespoon fat-free grated Parmesan cheese

1 medium slice French bread

1 teaspoon margarine

1 serving Banana-Caramel Pie (page 222)

Calories 565 • Fat 18g • Fiber 4g

SNACKS

1 serving Italian Salsa (page 34)

10 reduced-fat baked tortilla chips

Calories 75 • Fat 2g • Fiber 1g

TOTAL: CALORIES 1575 • FAT 32g • FIBER 20g

Calorie Chart

Food Item	Calories	Fat	Fiber
Beverages			
Alcoholic			
beer (8 ounces)	95	0	1
liquor (1 ounce)	65	0	0
mixed drinks (2.5 ounces)	140	0	0
wine (4 ounces)	80	0	0
Carbonated (8 ounces)			
cola	95	0	0
ginger ale	90	0	0
lemonade	90	0	0
sugar-free	0	0	0
tonic water	90	0	0
Coffee (8 ounces)			
black	5	0	0
with cream and sugar	40	2	0
Milk-type (8 ounces)			
cocoa with milk	140	4	1
eggnog, regular	305	17	0
eggnog, light	170	7	0
malted milk shake, chocolate	345	15	0
Milk			
buttermilk, skim	90	2	0
evaporated	305	17	0
low-fat, 2 percent	115	4	0
skim	80	0	0
whole	140	8	0
Tea (8 ounces)	0	0	0
Breads, Cereal and Grain Products			
Bagel (1 plain)	155	1	1
Biscuit (2-inch)	195	11	0
Breads (1-ounce slice raisin, white or whole wheat)	65	1	0
reduced-calorie, thinly sliced	40	1	0
Cereals			
Cooked (1/2 cup)			
cornmeal	65	0	1
cream of wheat	60	0	0
oatmeal	75	1	2

Food Item	Calories	Fat	Fiber
Breads, Cereal and Grain Products *(cont.)*			
Cereals *(cont.)*			
Dry			
Fiber One® (1/2 cup)	60	1	12
flaked cereal/ bran, corn and wheat (1 cup)	100	0	2
puffed cereal, rice and wheat (1 cup)	55	0	0
wheat, shredded (1 biscuit)	85	1	2
Cornbread (2-inch square)	130	5	1
Crackers			
graham (2 1/2-inch square)	30	1	0
saltine (2-inch square)	15	0	0
Croissant (1 plain)	325	19	1
Dried beans and lentils (1/2 cup cooked)	120	0	5
English muffin (1 plain)	135	1	1
Flour, all-purpose (1 tablespoon)	30	0	0
Muffin (2 1/2-inch)			
blueberry muffin	110	4	0
Pancake (4-inch)	75	1	0
Pasta (1/2 cup cooked)	100	0	1
Rice (1/2 cup cooked)	105	0	0
Rice cake (4-inch)	35	0	0
Rolls (1 average)			
hamburger or hot dog	125	2	1
hard	145	2	1
sweet	170	5	1
Tortilla, regular (8-inch)	140	3	1
Tortilla, fat-free	110	0	1
Waffle (4 1/2 × 3 3/4-inch)	90	3	0
Wheat germ (3 tablespoons)	80	2	3
Zwieback (1 piece)	30	1	0

(continues on next page)

Calorie Chart (cont.)

Food Item	Calories	Fat	Fiber
Cheese			
American, regular (1 ounce)	115	9	0
American, fat-free (1 ounce)	35	0	0
Cheddar, regular (1 ounce)	115	9	0
Cheddar, reduced-fat (1 ounce)	80	5	0
Cottage, regular (1/4 cup)	55	2	0
Cottage, low-fat (1/4 cup)	50	1	0
Cottage, nonfat (1/4 cup)	35	0	0
Cream, regular (1 ounce)	100	10	0
Neufchâtel (1 ounce)	60	5	0
Cream, nonfat (1 ounce)	25	0	0
Mozzarella, part-skim (1 ounce)	80	5	0
Parmesan (1 tablespoon grated)	25	2	0
Parmesan, fat-free grated (1 ounce)	105	0	0
Spread (1 ounce)	90	8	0
Swiss (1 ounce)	105	8	0
Desserts			
Apple Betty (1/2 cup)	303	11	3
Brownies (2 × 1-inch square)	110	10	0
Cake			
angel food (10-inch, 1/12, plain)	140	0	0
chocolate/chocolate icing (2-layer 1/16)	330	13	0
cupcake, plain (2 1/2-inch)	80	3	0
pound, fat-free (1/8 loaf)	120	0	0
pound (1/2-inch slice)	140	9	0
Cheesecake			
cake, from mix (1/8)	260	12	0
Cookies			
chocolate chip (2 1/3-inch)	100	5	0
ginger snap (1 1/2-inch)	25	1	0
oatmeal with raisins (2 3/4-inch)	80	3	0
sandwich (1 1/2-inch)	45	2	0
shortbread (1 1/2-inch square)	40	2	0
sugar (3-inch)	75	4	0
vanilla wafer (1 1/2-inch)	25	1	0
Custard (1/2 cup)	135	5	0
Doughnuts			
cake-type, plain	170	10	0
raised	240	14	1
raised, jelly center	335	17	1

Food Item	Calories	Fat	Fiber
Desserts *(cont.)*			
Eclair, custard filling, chocolate icing	280	17	0
Gelatin (1/2 cup)			
regular, fruit-flavored	80	0	0
sugar-free, fruit-flavored	10	0	0
Gingerbread (2-inch square)	205	7	0
Ice cream, vanilla (1/2 cup)			
premium	320	22	1
regular	135	7	0
fat-free	90	0	0
Ice milk, vanilla (1/2 cup)			
hardened	90	3	0
soft-serve	110	3	0
Pies (9-inch, 1/8)			
fruit, 2-crust	440	21	2
custard	275	14	0
lemon meringue	405	15	0
pecan	540	31	2
pumpkin	325	15	2
Pudding (1/2 cup)			
bread with raisins	210	8	1
chocolate, regular with whole milk	125	3	0
chocolate, sugar-free with skim milk	50	0	0
chocolate, fat-free, sugar-free	35	0	1
rice with raisins	185	3	0
tapioca	110	3	0
Sherbet (1/2 cup)	130	2	0
Shortcake, strawberry	205	9	2
Eggs (1 egg)			
Egg product, fat-free, cholesterol-free (1/4 cup)	25	0	0
Cooked, hard or soft	75	5	0
Fried or scrambled	110	8	0
Fats and Oils			
Butter (1 tablespoon)	100	12	0
Cream			
whipping (1 tablespoon)	45	5	0
sour (1 tablespoon)	30	3	0
coffee (1 tablespoon)	30	3	0
half-and-half (1 tablespoon)	20	2	0
half-and-half, fat-free (2 tablespoons)	10	0	0

Food Item	Calories	Fat	Fiber
Fats and Oils *(cont.)*			
Lard (1 tablespoon)	115	13	0
Margarine			
regular (1 tablespoon)	100	11	0
reduced-calorie (1 tablespoon)	50	6	0
Nonstick cooking spray	0	0	0
Oil, vegetable	120	14	0
Vegetable oil spread			
regular vegetable oil spread (1 tablespoon)	102	11	0
reduced-calorie vegetable oil spread (1 tablespoon)	70	8	0
nonfat vegetable oil spread (1 tablespoon)	5	0	0
Salad dressings (1 tablespoon)			
Blue cheese			
regular	75	8	0
reduced-calorie	15	0	0
French			
regular	65	6	0
reduced-calorie	35	3	0
Mayonnaise or salad dressing			
regular	100	11	0
reduced-calorie	50	5	0
fat-free	10	0	0
Ranch			
regular ranch	55	5	0
reduced-fat ranch	55	6	0
fat-free ranch	25	0	0
Thousand Island			
regular	60	6	0
reduced-calorie	25	2	0
Fruits and Fruit Juices			
Apple (2 3/4-inch)	80	0	4
Apple juice (1/2 cup)	60	0	0
Applesauce (1/2 cup)			
canned, sweetened	95	0	1
canned, unsweetened	50	0	1
Apricots			
canned, sweetened (1/2 cup)	80	0	1
canned, unsweetened (1/2 cup)	30	0	1
fresh (3 medium)	50	0	2
Avocado (1 slice)	15	2	0
Banana (7 inches)	85	0	2
Blackberries, fresh (1/2 cup)	35	0	3
Blueberries, fresh (1/2 cup)	40	0	2
Cantaloupe (5-inch, 1/2)	95	1	2

Food Item	Calories	Fat	Fiber
Fruits and Fruit Juices *(cont.)*			
Cherries			
canned, sweetened (1/2 cup)	90	1	2
canned, unsweetened (1/2 cup)	65	1	2
fresh (1/2 cup)	50	1	2
maraschino (1 large)	5	0	0
Coconut, shredded, firmly packed (1/2 cup)	235	17	2
Cranberry sauce, sweetened (1/2 cup)	215	0	1
Dates (3 medium)	70	0	2
Fig, dried (1 large)	50	0	2
Fruit cocktail, sweetened (1/2 cup)	70	0	1
Grapes, green seedless (1/2 cup)	55	0	1
Grape juice, canned (1/2 cup)	65	0	0
Grapefruit (1/2 medium)	45	0	1
Grapefruit juice, canned (1/2 cup)	65	0	0
Honeydew melon (5-inch, 1/4)	55	0	1
Lemon juice (1 tablespoon)	5	0	0
Nectarine (2-inch)	65	0	2
Orange (medium)	60	0	3
Orange juice, unsweetened (1/2 cup)	55	0	0
Peach			
canned, sweetened (1/2 cup)	70	0	1
canned, unsweetened (1/2 cup)	30	0	1
fresh (1 medium)	35	0	2
Pear			
canned, sweetened (1/2 cup)	95	0	2
canned, unsweetened (1/2 cup)	35	0	1
fresh (2 1/2-inch, medium)	100	1	4
Pineapple			
canned, sweetened (1 large slice)	80	0	1
juice, unsweetened (1/2 cup)	70	0	0
fresh (1/2 cup)	40	0	1
Plum, fresh (2 1/8-inch, medium)	35	0	1
Prunes (4 medium)	80	0	2
Prune juice (1/2 cup)	91	0	1
Pumpkin, canned (1/2 cup)	40	0	3
Raisins, dry (2 tablespoons)	60	0	1
Raspberries, fresh (1/2 cup)	30	0	4

(continues on next page)

Calorie Chart (cont.)

Food Item	Calories	Fat	Fiber
Fruits and Fruit Juices *(cont.)*			
Rhubarb, stewed, sweetened			
(1/2 cup)	140	0	2
Strawberries (1/2 cup)			
fresh	25	0	2
frozen, sweetened	120	0	2
Tangerine (2 1/2-inch)	35	0	2
Watermelon (10 × 1-inch slice)	155	2	2
Meats (lean, well-trimmed, 3 ounces cooked)			
Beef			
chuck	210	13	0
corned	215	13	0
Ground beef			
regular	260	19	0
lean	244	17	0
extra-lean	210	13	0
Liver, fried	185	7	0
Roast			
rib	210	13	0
rump	155	4	0
Steak			
flank	175	8	0
porterhouse	175	8	0
round	155	4	0
sirloin	153	4	0
tenderloin beef	175	8	0
T-bone	175	8	0
Lamb			
chop, loin	175	8	0
roast			
leg	175	8	0
shoulder	175	8	0
Pork			
chop, loin	180	9	0
Ham			
cured	150	8	0
fresh	180	9	0
Roast, loin	180	9	0
Tenderloin	140	4	0
Veal			
chop, loin	140	5	0
cutlet	140	5	0
roast	140	5	0
Miscellaneous			
turkey bacon (2 slices)	60	4	0
bacon (2 medium slices)	75	6	0

Food Item	Calories	Fat	Fiber
Meats *(cont.)*			
bologna (4 1/2 × 1/8-inch slice)	90	8	0
Braunschweiger			
(2 × 1/4-inch slice)	35	3	0
hot dog (1 regular)	145	13	0
hot dogs, reduced-fat (1)	140	11	0
hot dogs, fat-free (1)	45	0	0
pork link (3 × 1/2-inch)	50	4	0
Nuts			
Almonds (1/4 cup)	210	19	4
Brazil (4)	105	11	1
Cashews (1/4 cup)	185	16	1
Hazelnuts (6)	55	5	0
Peanuts, reduced-fat (1/4 cup)	115	8	0
Peanuts (1/4 cup)	210	18	3
Pecans (1/4 cup)	180	18	2
Walnuts (1/4 cup)	160	15	1
Poultry (3 ounces cooked)			
Chicken			
breast, broiled	140	3	0
breast, fried, with bone	228	13	0
drumstick, fried, with bone	274	17	0
ground	155	5	0
roasted, no skin	155	5	0
Goose, roasted, no skin	185	10	0
Turkey			
breast slices	140	3	0
roasted, no skin	155	5	0
tenderloins	140	3	0
ground	200	12	0
breast, ground	140	3	0
Sauces (2 tablespoons)			
Butterscotch	105	0	0
Cheese	65	5	0
Chili	30	0	0
Chocolate	80	0	0
Hollandaise	90	9	0
Lemon curd	100	2	0
Tartar, regular	150	16	0
Tartar, fat-free	25	0	0
Tomato	10	0	0
White	50	3	0

Food Item	Calories	Fat	Fiber
Seafood (3 ounces)			
Clams, canned	125	2	0
Cod, broiled	100	1	0
Crabmeat, canned	85	1	0
Fish stick, batter-dipped	200	10	0
Halibut, broiled	100	1	0
Lobster, canned	85	1	0
Oysters, raw	60	2	0
Salmon, pink, canned	120	5	0
Sardines, canned in oil	175	10	0
Scallops, steamed	100	1	0
Shrimp			
canned	85	1	0
French fried	235	15	0
Tuna			
canned in oil	170	7	0
water-packed	100	1	0
Soups (made with water, 1 cup)			
Bean with pork	170	6	9
Beef noodle	85	3	1
Bouillon	30	0	0
Clam chowder	90	3	1
Cream of chicken	115	7	0
Cream of chicken, reduced-fat	140	4	0
Cream of mushroom	130	10	0
Cream of mushroom, reduced-fat	140	6	2
Oyster stew	85	2	1
Split pea	165	3	3
Tomato	180	4	2
Tomato, reduced-fat	85	2	0
Vegetable-beef	85	3	1
Sweets			
Candies			
caramel (1 medium)	30	1	0
chocolate			
bar, plain (1 ounce)	145	9	1
kisses (7)	175	10	1
fudge (1-inch square)	85	2	0
gumdrops (1 large or 8 small)	40	0	0
jelly beans (10)	100	0	0
lollipop (2 1/4-inch)	80	0	0
marshmallow (1 large)	25	0	0
peanut brittle (2 1/2-inch piece)	70	4	0

Food Item	Calories	Fat	Fiber
Sweets *(cont.)*			
Jams			
regular (1 tablespoon)	50	0	0
reduced-sugar (1 tablespoon)	45	0	1
Jellies			
regular (1 tablespoon)	45	0	0
reduced-sugar (1 tablespoon)	30	0	0
Preserves			
regular (1 tablespoon)	50	0	0
reduced-sugar (1 tablespoon)	45	0	1
Syrups			
chocolate-flavored (1 tablespoon)	40	0	0
hot fudge ice cream topping, fat-free (2 tablespoons)	110	0	0
caramel ice cream topping, fat-free (2 tablespoons)	130	0	0
corn (1 tablespoon)	60	0	0
honey (1 tablespoon)	65	0	0
maple (1 tablespoon)	50	0	0
maple-flavored, light (2 tablespoons)	15	0	0
molasses (1 tablespoon)	55	0	0
Sugars (1/2 cup)			
brown	415	0	0
granulated	385	0	0
powdered	235	0	0
Vegetables			
Asparagus, cooked (1/2 cup)	25	0	2
Bamboo shoots (1/2 cup)	10	0	2
Beans (1/2 cup)			
baked, no pork	125	1	6
green, cooked	20	0	2
kidney, cooked	115	0	6
lima, cooked	85	0	6
Bell pepper, raw (1 medium)	20	0	1
Beets, cooked (1/2 cup)	35	0	1
Beet greens, cooked (1/2 cup)	15	0	2
Broccoli, cooked (1/2 cup)	25	0	3
Brussels sprouts, cooked (1/2 cup)	35	0	4
Cabbage (1/2 cup)			
cooked	15	0	2
raw	10	0	1

(continues on next page)

Calorie Chart (cont.)

Food Item	Calories	Fat	Fiber
Vegetables *(cont.)*			
Carrots, cooked (1/2 cup)	35	0	2
Cauliflower, cooked (1/2 cup)	15	0	2
Celery (8 × 1/2-inch stalk)	5	0	0
Corn			
canned, whole kernel (1/2 cup)	65	1	1
cob (5 × 1 3/4-inch ear)	85	1	2
Cucumber (1/2 cup)	5	0	0
Eggplant, raw (1/2 cup)	10	0	1
Kale, cooked (1/2 cup)	20	0	2
Lettuce, iceberg (1/8 wedge, medium head)	10	0	1
Mushrooms, canned (1/4 cup)	10	0	1
Okra, cooked (3 × 5/8-inch, 8 pods)	30	0	2
Onions			
cooked (1/2 cup)	45	0	1
green (6 small)	30	0	2
Parsnips, cooked (1/2 cup)	65	0	3
Peas, cooked (1/2 cup)	60	0	4
Potato			
baked (2 1/4-inch)	85	0	1
French fried (2 × 1/2 inch, 10 pieces)	130	7	1
sweet (1/2 cup)	90	0	2
Radishes (4 small)	1	0	0
Rutabagas, cooked (1/2 cup)	35	0	1
Sauerkraut (1/2 cup)	20	0	3
Spinach, cooked (1/2 cup)	25	0	3
Squash, cooked (1/2 cup)			
summer	20	0	1
winter	55	0	3
Tomato			
canned (1/2 cup)	25	0	1
fresh (3-inch)	40	0	2
Tomato juice (1/2 cup)	20	0	0
Turnips, cooked (1/2 cup)	15	0	1
Water chestnuts (4)	15	0	0

Food Item	Calories	Fat	Fiber
Miscellaneous			
Catsup, regular (1 tablespoon)	15	0	0
Catsup, light (1 tablespoon)	10	0	0
Cocoa (1 tablespoon)	10	1	2
Chocolate, baking (1 ounce)	150	16	4
Gelatin, unflavored (1 envelope)	25	0	0
Gelatin pop, frozen	25	0	0
Gravy (1 tablespoon)	10	0	0
Gravy, low-fat (1 tablespoon)	5	0	0
Herring, pickled (1 × 1/2-inch)	40	3	0
Ice cream bar, chocolate-covered	180	13	0
Mustard, prepared (1 teaspoon)	5	0	0
Olives			
green (4 medium)	20	2	0
ripe (3 small)	10	1	0
Peanut butter (1 tablespoon)	95	8	1
Peanut butter spread, reduced-fat (1 tablespoon)	95	6	0
Pickles			
dill (3 3/4 × 1 1/4 inch)	10	0	1
relish (1 tablespoon)	20	0	0
sweet (2 1/2-inch × 3/4-inch)	20	0	0
Pizza, cheese (14-inch, 1/8)	235	7	1
Popcorn	30	0	1
added oil (1 cup)	105	9	1
microwave 94 percent fat-free (6 cups)	110	2	4
hot-air-popped (1 cup)	30	0	1
Popsicle	65	0	0
Potato chips (10)	110	7	1
Potato chips, low-fat (10)	84	4	1
Potato chips, fat-free (10)	35	0	2
Pretzels (3 inches, 5 sticks)	10	0	0
Pretzels, fat-free (1.1 ounces)	110	0	0
Vinegar (2 tablespoons)	5	0	0
Yeast, dry, active (1 package)	20	0	2
Yogurt (1 cup)			
made from whole milk	150	8	0
low-fat plain	155	4	0
nonfat plain	135	0	0

Source: General Mills, Inc.

Metric Conversion Guide

Volume

U.S. Units	Canadian Metric	Australian Metric
1/4 teaspoon	1 mL	1 ml
1/2 teaspoon	2 mL	2 ml
1 teaspoon	5 mL	5 ml
1 tablespoon	15 mL	20 ml
1/4 cup	50 mL	60 ml
1/3 cup	75 mL	80 ml
1/2 cup	125 mL	125 ml
2/3 cup	150 mL	170 ml
3/4 cup	175 mL	190 ml
1 cup	250 mL	250 ml
1 quart	1 liter	1 liter
1 1/2 quarts	1.5 liters	1.5 liters
2 quarts	2 liters	2 liters
2 1/2 quarts	2.5 liters	2.5 liters
3 quarts	3 liters	3 liters
4 quarts	4 liters	4 liters

Weight

U.S. Units	Canadian Metric	Australian Metric
1 ounce	30 grams	30 grams
2 ounces	55 grams	60 grams
3 ounces	85 grams	90 grams
4 ounces (1/4 pound)	115 grams	125 grams
8 ounces (1/2 pound)	225 grams	225 grams
16 ounces (1 pound)	455 grams	500 grams
1 pound	455 grams	1/2 kilogram

Note: The recipes in this cookbook have not been developed or tested using metric measures. When converting recipes to metric, some variations in quality may be noted.

Measurements

Inches	Centimeters
1	2.5
2	5.0
3	7.5
4	10.0
5	12.5
6	15.0
7	17.5
8	20.5
9	23.0
10	25.5
11	28.0
12	30.5
13	33.0
14	35.5
15	38.0

Temperatures

Fahrenheit	Celsius
32°	0°
212°	100°
250°	120°
275°	140°
300°	150°
325°	160°
350°	180°
375°	190°
400°	200°
425°	220°
450°	230°
475°	240°
500°	260°

Helpful Nutrition and Cooking Information

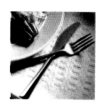

Nutrition Guidelines:

Daily Values are set by the Food and Drug Administration and are based on the needs of most healthy adults. Percent Daily Values are based on an average diet of 2,000 calories per day. Your daily values may be higher or lower depending on your calorie needs.

Recommended intake for a daily diet of 2,000 calories:

Total Fat	Less than 65 g
Saturated Fat	Less than 20 g
Cholesterol	Less than 300 mg
Sodium	Less than 2,400 mg
Total Carbohydrate	300 g
Dietary Fiber	25 g

Criteria Used for Calculating Nutrition Information:

- The first ingredient is used wherever a choice is given (such as 1/3 cup sour cream or plain yogurt).

- The first ingredient amount is used wherever a range is given (such as 2 to 3 teaspoons milk).

- The first serving number is used wherever a range is given (such as 4 to 6 servings).

- "If desired" ingredients are not included, whether mentioned in the ingredient list or in the recipe directions as a suggestion (such as sprinkle with brown sugar if desired).

- Only the amount of a marinade or frying oil that is absorbed during preparation is calculated.

Cooking Terms Glossary:

Beat: Make smooth with a vigorous stirring motion using a spoon, wire whisk, egg beater or electric mixer.

Boil: Heat liquid until bubbles keep rising and breaking on the surface.

Chop: Cot food into small, uneven pieces; a sharp knife, food chopper or food processor may be used.

Core: Cut out the stem end and remove the seeds.

Cut in: Mix fat into a flour mixture with a pastry blender with a rolling motion or cutting with a fork or two knives until particles are size specified.

Dice: Cut into cubes smaller than 1/2 inch.

Drain: Pour off liquid or let it run off through the holes in a strainer or colander, as when draining cooked pasta or ground beef. Or, remove pieces of food from a fat or liquid and set them on paper towels to soak up excess moisture.

Flute: Flatten pastry evenly on rim of pie plate and press firmly around rim with tines of fork.

Grate: Rub against small holes of grater to cut into tiny pieces.

Grease: Spread the bottoms and side of a disk or pan with solid vegetable shortening using a pastry brush or paper towel.

Knead: Curve your fingers and fold dough toward you, then push it away with the heels of your hands, using a quick rocking motion.

Mix: combine to distribute ingredients evenly using a spoon, fork, blender or an electric mixer.

Peel: Cut off the skin with a knife or peel with fingers.

Pipe: Press out frosting from a decorating bag using steady pressure to form a design or write a message. To finish a design, stop the pressure and lift the pint up and away.

Roll or **Pat:** Flatten and spread with a floured rolling pin or hands.

Ingredients used in recipe testing and nutrition calculations:

- Large eggs, canned ready-to-use chicken broth, 2% milk, 80%-lean ground beef and vegetable-oil spread with at least 65% fat. These are used as they are the most commonly purchased ingredients within those categories.

- Regular long-grain white rice wherever cooked rice is listed, unless indicated.

- Nonfat, low-fat or low-sodium products are not used, unless indicated.

- Solid vegetable shortening (not margarine, butter and nonstick cooking sprays, as they can cause sticking problems) us used to grease pans, unless indicated.

Equipment used in Recipe Testing:

- Cookware and bakeware *without* nonstick coatings are used, unless indicated.

- Wherever a baking *pan* is specified in a recipe, a *metal* pan is used; wherever a baking *dish* or pie *plate* is specified, ovenproof *glass* or *ceramic* ovenware is used.

- A portable electric hand mixer is used for mixing *only when mixer speeds are specified* in the recipe directions.

Low-Fat Shopping and Stocking

Shopping Smart Tips

- Shop for groceries after you've eaten, instead of when you are hungry—you'll be less vulnerable.

- Less time spent in the supermarket means less temptation time. Prepare a shopping list and try to stick to it.

- Avoid using coupons for high-fat or novelty items—they may cost you more in the long run!

- Buy lower-fat foods that you love and that will set you for success, not sabotage you once you get them home.

- Educate yourself on reading food labels so that you can use them to comparison shop.

- Be aware. Food items with more than 3 grams of fat per 100 calories have more than 30% of calories coming from fat.

- While waiting in line to check out, glance over the food in your cart and remove any item that may tempt you once you get home.

The Fish and Poultry Sections

- Turkey and chicken franks are not necessarily low in fat. Check their food labels.

- Half of chicken's calories are in the skin. Buy skinless parts or remove skin before cooking.

- For the leanest ground turkey available, buy ground turkey breast. Most butchers will grind it for you.

- Shellfish contains less fat than does meat or poultry.

- Limit fowl such as duck and goose, which are extremely high in fat.

The Meat Counter

- "Prime" grades of meat are heavily marbled with fat, making them a higher-fat choice.

- Select lean cuts of beef, such as round steak, sirloin tip, tenderloin and extra-lean ground beef.

- Select lean pork, such as tenderloin, loin chops, center-cut ham and Canadian bacon.

- Wild game, such as buffalo, venison, rabbit, squirrel and pheasant, are very lean.

The Dairy Case

- Plain nonfat yogurt is high in protein and calcium and can help replace mayonnaise in salads and dips.

- A little sharp cheese adds more flavor and less fat than a larger amount of milder cheese.

- Buttermilk is low in fat despite its name. It's made from cultured skim milk.

The Produce Section

- Purchase extra fresh vegetables to chop and add to purchased deli salads.

- Approach fruits and vegetables with reckless abandon. With the exception of avocados, they both are virtually fat-free.

- Marinate frozen vegetable mixes (without sauce) in reduced-calorie Italian dressing.

- Frozen fruit and juice bars can satisfy a sweet craving without the fat found in ice cream.

20 Pantry Pleasers

These foods make a big impact in flavor, but not in fat. Keep them on hand in your pantry.

1. **Reduced-calorie Italian dressing:** Great for marinating raw vegetables or as a dressing for cold potatoes or pasta salad.

2. **Salsa:** With only 20 calories and less than 1 gram of fat per 1/4 cup, salsa is perfect to top potatoes or serve with chicken and fish.

3. **Spaghetti/pasta sauce:** Use to make spaghetti, lasagne and manicotti, or toss with garden vegetables and serve over pasta.

4. **Stewed/chopped tomatoes:** Use as base for tomato sauces, soups or chili. Now available in Mexican, Italian and Cajun-style varieties.

5. **Canned chopped chilies:** With seeds and membranes removed, these chilies are mild in flavor but an excellent enhancement to most any Mexican food.

6. **Canned beans:** High in fiber and practically fat-free, beans are a great item to have on hand. Try a variety in soups, salads or puréed in blender for vegetarian pâté.

7. **Canned evaporated skimmed milk:** Great substitute for half-and-half in cream sauces and soups or can be reconstituted and used in recipes calling for skim milk.

8. **Pasta and rice:** Cooks in minutes with lots of variety and wide appeal. Brown rice and whole wheat pasta have the added benefit of being a rich source of fiber.

9. **Sesame oil:** This oil has a deliciously nutty taste. It does have the calories and fat of oil, but you need only a very little to boost the flavor in salads and stir-frys.

10. **Seasoned rice vinegar:** Made from fermented rice and sugar, this vinegar (typically used in sushi) makes fabulous salad dressing. Look for it in the oriental section of your grocery store.

11. **Chicken broth (dry):** Convenient for recipes calling for chicken broth. Look for crystals, cubes or individual packets that do not contain fat in the ingredient list.

12. **Assorted dried herbs and spices** (dill, oregano, basil, chili powder, cumin, curry): Flavor foods as mildly or intensely as you desire without adding fat or calories.

13. **Garlic:** A wonderfully aromatic addition to most any food! Buy it by the bulb or prepared in a jar (1/2 teaspoon equals 1 clove). Store bulbs in a cool place.

14. **Lemons:** Fresh lemon adds flavor without fat to plain or seltzer water. Lemon also enhances prepared salad dressing, fish and fresh cooked vegetables.

15. **Fresh gingerroot:** Grated or chopped, this tropical root adds a wonderfully complex flavor to stir-frys and marinades. Refrigerate up to a week or wrap and keep in freezer up to 2 months.

16. **Grated Parmesan cheese:** A great bargain at 23 calories per tablespoon (1 1/2 grams of fat). Use on popcorn, pasta, fish, soup and baked potatoes.

17. **Fat-free egg product:** Made mostly out of egg whites, a good substitute for whole eggs in baked products and omelets. It's also nice to have on hand when you run out of eggs!

18. **Nonfat dairy products** (milk, yogurt, sour cream, cottage cheese): Excellent as a substitute for higher fat varieties; great source of protein and calcium.

19. **Frozen berries:** Add to muffins and pancake batter; mix with yogurt and juice in blender; purée for dessert topping; or eat as a snack right out of the freezer.

20. **Frozen chopped spinach:** A wonderful addition to soups, lasagne, pizza and dips, and an excellent source of iron, vitamin C and beta carotene.

Index

Numbers in *italics* refer to photographs.